WRITERS CROSSING BOUNDARIES:
Writing the Real World

Deborah M. Coulter-Harris, Ph.D
The University of Toledo

Linus
Publications, Inc.

Published by Linus Publications, Inc.

Deer Park, NY 11729

ISBN 1-934188-77-8

Printed in the United States of America.

10 9 8 7 6 5 4 3 2 1

Writers Crossing Boundaries:
First Edition

Dr. Deborah Coulter-Harris

This book should appeal to composition students, writing and literature instructors, and the general reading public. I have tried to integrate my own writing experiences to show how many diverse and exciting opportunities exist for writers in varied fields and locations.

The Book's Featured Inclusions

- The **author's personal experiences** writing for radio, corporations, the military, and the CIA.

- **Part I, Writing the Real World, includes 12 Pyramid steps to Writing Analysis and Research:** section contains a logical process for teaching students to conduct research and explore analytic writing.

- **Appendices** include evaluation forms for individual research projects, several analytic techniques, and analytic methods examples.

- **Samples of author's creative writing**: poetry, literary analysis, political analysis, and satire.

- **Diverse array of readings in Part II** includes: political science readings, American poetry, British and Irish poetry, Satire, and readings on religion. Each reading section contains writing prompts for use in the writing classroom arena, or for use by avid readers and creative thinkers.

TABLE OF CONTENTS

PART I

Writing The Real World

PART II

Reading & Writing Memories

SECTION I

SECTION IV

SECTION V

PART I

WRITING FOR THE REAL WORLD

Preface to Writing

18 July, 2006
Dear Readers,

I had no idea when I began to write a 10 to 20 page essay in collaboration with an academic colleague that this manuscript would blossom into over 500 pages. I hope my readers feel entertained and inspired by my thoughts about my life travels, and my life experiences as a writer for the corporate, military, and CIA; I further hope the readings and literary commentary will amuse my readers in the second part of this book. I hope to write many more of these types of books, for I have much to say and much to report on about world conditions and about the human condition. Enjoy the book.

Dr. Deborah Coulter-Harris

Introduction

Letter from Dr. Carol Nelson-Burns

April, 2006
Dear Deb,

Having just returned from, and been once again inspired by, CCCC presentations and discussions, I am writing to enlist your participation in a new project conceived in Chicago. To my delight, one of the newest movements in the field of composition studies is a call for what has been coined "creative non-fiction." Loosely defined as memoir or travel writing, among other titles and topics, this new branching seems at first to contradict our efforts to guide "basic writers'" propensity to narrate and describe all information into the more highly prized "analytic" writing that has been the hallmark of "critical thinking." However, somewhere along the way it seems that the authentic voice has been lost; the press for the more impersonal voice bolstered by unbiased research studies has led us into a vapid collection of meaningless statistics, figures, data. The latter documents are often heartless, soul-less, sterile—and monotonously similar. Most of us don't recall the last good statistic we read.

An examination of the state of the academy's regard for and practical use of traditionally valued professorial productivity will help underscore the need for embracing "creative non-fiction" as a viable contribution to "new knowledge" in our profession. To that end, I have identified colleagues whose unique experiences and perspectives can make an important contribution to this discussion. I am asking you to contribute the following to the longer discussion I am envisioning:

Professionals Developing: Race, Gender, and Class Valued and Voiced
Deborah Coulter-Harris: "Publishing in the Profession, and Writing for Real"

What I have in mind is a 5-20 page discussion drawing from YOUR experiences (anecdotal accepted) and your professional life (memoirs, biographic, etc). Specifically, I have heard the English dept. "colleagues" evaluate each others' writings, looking at some publication as that of a real "scholar" and typically de-valuing the kind of writing done in the field by which the lives of others are enriched in a way that a scholarly journal article fails. I'd like you to talk about your experiences writing in government circles, PDRs?—not revealing what you said or didn't, but the process you went through to write such things, the impact of such writing, and the ultimate value of THAT kind of writing as the illusive "new knowledge" which uni profs argue THEIR work is all about...

I am hoping to bring this material together by late summer and would appreciate receiving a substantial draft version by early June.

Many thanks!!
Carol Nelson-Burns

Writers Crossing Boundaries: Where Paths Take You[1]

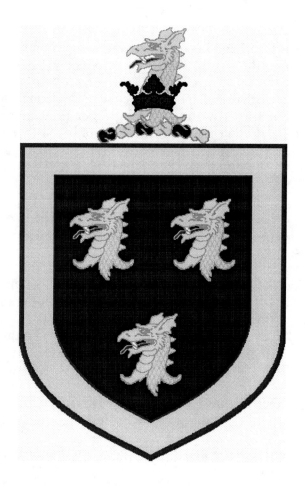

Dr. Deborah M. Coulter-Harris

---

1 The above shield is the Scottish Coulter crest.

By Dr. Deborah M. Coulter-Harris

May 2006

Dear Carol:

I am happy to respond to your above proposal. I will, of course, have to send my drafts to the Central Intelligence Agency (CIA) for clearance before providing anyone with a draft (see Appendix 2 for request for review letters). I hope this letter responds to recent writing theories that I thought were too self-absorbed and not able to bring us into the new global economy. We in the future will rely on other nations to provide goods and services to us, which may not be so politically sound, but it's already reality. We've given up too much land and industry to foreigners, who may or may not have larger designs on our united territories. Our writing students will face greater global challenges than ever my generation did growing up.

I don't know exactly where this manuscript will go in addressing your suggested inclusions of my writing and life experiences thereof. In terms of my memories of my writing profession, there is much to tell about creative sides and professional sides. My writing experiences at times derived from people I met in my many travels, and have had enchanted encounters with Irish fisherman and sheep farmers and people of royalty. I have met and studied with soldiers, and once was myself a soldier. I met actors and directors and CEOs of corporations. I also met many Greek people near the Aegean, and studied Torah with Conservative Jews in Philadelphia. I studied with many professors here and abroad, and have studied with an international array of priests, rabbis, and ministers of the Gospel. I never studied with an Imam, but I have read the Koran two or three times, and taught about Islam in a comparative religion composition class in Philadelphia and New Jersey (see Appendix 3 for a list of web resources on religious conflicts). This is just a partial list of my encounters—I have lived. Most lately, I worked with the men down at CIA, and met many people in our government and military. I liked working for CIA, but I would rather have a permanent home up North, where I'm from.

Memory Animates Analysis

Memory is the accumulation of sensory experience and should not be limited to ordinary personal narratives at a university level. Memory makes writing possible through research and study of a multitude of disciplines; the ability to remember information and apply that data quickly to analysis is the number one demand of the marketplace. Memory is who we are as people, the memory of our ancestors and the connections we have with others and the connections we do not. I am my memories of travels, of scholarship, of very hard work; everything I am as a writer includes my environment, but cultural considerations do not surpass accumulation of knowledge and experience and bits of wisdom learned. I like to connect the images I have seen and heard and studied and tried to make *image connections* with other cultures, religions, politics, economies, militaries; I want to understand how people and nations connect, our ancient origins, the truth of who we all are and who we are not.

A writer/analyst's memory is central to the analytic process; memory is not just the aptitude to recollect facts, but to recall patterns that relate factors to broader concepts.

"According to Plato, human perception reveals phenomena as transient or relative surface reality, whereas reason detects an absolute, permanent, universal, homogeneous reality….Sensory objects exist in the perceptual, world, while the principles of reality exist in the metaphysical world of thought" (Sahakian 125).

As an analyst, I have learned through experience that I do not want to perceive what I expect to perceive. Patterns of expectation become so ingrained that they actuate perceptions—being "objective" does not ensure accurate discernment and, consequently, sound analysis. My experiences and education can impair my analysis; writer/analysts are prone to assimilate ambiguous data into pre-existing ideas that validate entrenched views. For example, what is your perception of the image below in figure 1? Is it first of a young woman or an old woman? If you see a young woman, are you having difficulty perceiving the image of the old woman because of some type of *resistance*?[2] This is what analysis requires: to study information and reorganize it visually or mentally, to apprehend it from a contrary perspective. Perspective once formed resists other outlooks.

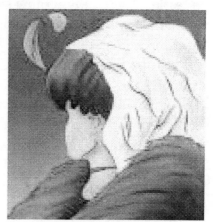

Figure 1. "My Wife and My Mother-In-Law"

2　This picture was originally published in Puck magazine in 1915, and was entitled "My Wife and My Mother-In-Law."

All writing involves memory: *creative writing* remembers symbols and images and makes them fun to read and think about and connect to and be part of; *professional and business writing* remembers contracts, old and new, remembers proposals, and promotes the United States' economy; *classical argument* remembers laws and promotes structure and order of thinking and rational thought (see Appendix 4 for notes on classical thinkers).

Creative Non-Fiction as Original Scholarship

I see what you refer to *"creative non-fiction"* is the type of writing that occurs at the highest echelons of corporate society, government, and the military [three bulks of my writing memories—the other bulk creative] where it is their charge to analyze the world and secure United States' preeminence. I am certainly behind that idea, for I would resist any encroachment on this land. This type of writing requires deep creativity.

"Creative non-fiction" is your arrival as a writer, who has accumulated the expertise to create theories without referring to Moses and his brother Aaron and every other theorist who ever lived in Moscow. Creative non-fiction comes from experience in the field, writing for the real world, *writing for real.* I guess what I'm trying to say is that I am writing this manuscript from *"knowing"* and not much from further reference or research than is needed. I am *remembering* all that has been taught to me in my life about writing, including all literary and political theories from Aristotle to Derrida, but I also have my own *reconstituted views*[3] on writing. I sincerely hope that *I may be my writing* in this book, wherever patterns lead us this summer, 2006.

The highest paying and most interesting jobs today for university graduates are with global corporations and companies, entities that demand the writing skills I describe. Certainly my experiences as a Middle East political analyst at CIA demanded only the very best writing and analysis for the President and his Cabinet; analyst writers are carefully appointed—these are selective positions, and you do bear influence. Standards of dress and behavior are strict, and your life is closely monitored and secured; you don't have much of a social life.

I know from serving as a Russian translator for US Army Intelligence that writing for the military requires the same technical skills, and these writing competencies are copied by the civilian corporate world. The military, of course, demands strict precision in collection, translation, and analysis; my experience for U.S. Military Intelligence consisted of laborious translations of Soviet military documents in the 1980s at the Command and General Staff College at Fort Leavenworth. This happened directly upon returning to the United

---

3   I am using the adjective "reconstituted" with reference to more classical roots but with change.

States from Greece, where I had lived for one year with the United States Army at a former NATO nuclear site in northern Greece; it was dismantled during the last month of my stay. I left just a few months before the Chernobyl My professional writing life began at MOSTEK Corporation in Dallas, Texas: served as technical writer for semiconductor standards, supervisor of largely Vietnamese employees in Burn-In[4], and then Speech Writer and Executive Assistant (E.A.) to Mr.L. J. Sevin, MOSTEK's founder.[5] Earlier in my life, shortly after receiving my B.A., I lived in England and was administrative assistant to a retired Colonel in the British Army, and was English instructor at the same British utility company.

As E.A. to L.J. Sevin, I had my own office, and I was included in quarterly and annual meetings in Dallas, and had the opportunity to attend a two-day meeting with United Technologies (UT) corporate big-wigs during the sale of Mostek to UT at Mostek's[6] headquarters in Carrollton, Texas, in 1980. I attended meetings where Alexander Haig was present, as were many automobile executives. I enjoyed working for L.J. Sevin; he would most times give me four words to base a briefing on. I spent most of my time analyzing projected quarterly goals versus actual profits. I taught a speech course, and wrote L.J.'s speeches.

In the mid-1980s I spent a year with my husband attached to a NATO nuclear base in the northern town of Drama, Greece. I taught United States History and English Composition to U.S. soldiers serving at the base, and taught English in the evenings at a private *Anglika*, an English training school. *Phillipi*, the location of Paul's imprisonment, was only a short ten minutes drive from Drama; I was surprised how low the thresholds were in the ancient ruins, and I imaged *Lilliputian* people living back then. I much enjoyed the northern beaches of the Aegean and learned to snorkel, and I began to resemble a Spaniard.

Although I hold a Ph.D. in British Literature and Linguistics, all of my best professional writing jobs were in the realms spoken above. What is thrilling about this type of writing is it requires as much creativity as artistic writing: analyzing patterns of thought, creating solutions to real life problems, having influence with policy makers etc.—a not so different world than writing within the Academy, just on a real secret stage.

Writing Standards at CIA

There's been a lot of bad news lately about the CIA, mostly unfounded and bitterly political. People should not be shocked to know that the Directorate of

---

4   The Burn-In stage electrifies semiconductors.

5   I worked for L. J. just before he sold his company to United Technologies during General Alexander Haig's tenure as its President.

6   Mostek owned plants in Ireland and in Taiwan, and employed thousands of people in the Dallas area.

Intelligence (DI) requires its writer analysts to possess first-class writing skills because its analysis has proven to be best in the world, despite vital lapses of HUMINT [Human Intelligence] information from the field (but that was due to budget). CIA's analysts pursue a rigorous six months at the Sherman Kent[7] School of Analysis (see Appendix 5); some quit in the first six months because of the intellectual and psychological rigors at Kent. Most writer analysts have an M.A. or a Ph.D. and possess skills that are vital to our nation; most of these folk come from the Ivy League, but CIA is also open to people who have cumulative skills in many academic disciplines. Analytic tradecraft is as creative as any art; my training in literary analysis in the University of Toledo's Ph.D. program was perfect in preparing me for analytic work at CIA (see Appendix 6 for a sample of literary analysis with writing assignments). I think the Agency should become more vital with an older, more diverse workforce. The DI needs the smarts of many of our more experienced professors, people who already are accomplished thinkers. Also, I don't think that the United States' CIA is a southern agency, is it?

Competition at CIA

CIA analysts are very competitive in publications, as are academics at universities. The highest publication an analyst can achieve is the PDB (Presidential Daily Brief) (see Appendix 7) and I published several; only the President and a very small number of people read this publication. Analysts at CIA can receive kudos from the President and other policy makers, and can earn extra monetary awards for their success. The next type of publication is a SEIB (Senior Executive Intelligence Brief), which the President and a slightly wider audience reads on a daily basis; I was a SEIB machine on many topics of global concern. Analysts complete every day for this publication. Longer papers, IAs (Intelligence Assessments), are identical to university research scholarship with the exception of added classified intelligence; at least half or more of my writing at CIA consisted of IAs. There are *also National Intelligence Estimates* (NIE) that predict larger issues in the future, and everyone at Agency coordinates on that publication.

My training as a Russian linguist at the Defense Language Center, Foreign Language Center (DLIFLC) in Monterey, California, was first rate. Students are immersed in languages to the extent I eventually had problems writing English letters after nearly two years of study. My teachers at DLI were primary from the old Soviet Union; we had a brain surgeon from the USSR's old army, and he used to fall asleep in class— most of them drank vodka on the weekends. An ex-Soviet

---

7 Sherman Kent worked in the Research and Analysis branch of the OSS (Office of Strategic Services) during World War II and is famous for his treatise, *Strategic Intelligence for American World Power*; Kent revered the analyst.

journalist said every day during lab time that, ""I veel not keel you tooo-day, maybe tomorrow, but not tooo-day." While living in the Monterey area, I performed as the Wife of Bath in the rock musical version of *Canterbury Tales* at the Forest Theatre in Carmel just before going to Greece. I would encourage students to find an outlet to develop an artistic side—makes them better rounded and more of an extrovert. I was one of few extroverts in the DI at CIA.

The Psychology of Words

I often warn people to be careful what you say, because the words you use create your circumstance: for example, do we continue to trust people whose words are rarely true, and live in their reality; or, do we create a new reality by the words we choose? I like to remember the ancient prophets and the words they spoke on the Lord's behalf to the people of Israel, and I like to evaluate the predictive words they spoke and how faithfully their words came true.

I like getting to the root of words, and learning its ancient origins. For example, the *Anakim* of the Hebrew Bible originates in *ante-deluvian Sumerian culture*, with the arrival of the *Annunaki*, the ancient *dragon gods*, the men spoken of in Genesis, those from the sky who came down and mated with human woman to produce a race of giants. The descendants of these "angels" were the giants Joshua and his men saw in Canaan before the Hebrew invasion. These giants and dragons are characters in almost every ancient literature around the globe, especially in northern countries, and other more southerly countries like Italy and Greece.

I have learned that my words have a deep impact on people I know, and for that reason, I like to speak words of kindness to my friends and loved ones. I have also become aware that if I continue to hold myself in low-esteem, I would create the reality that others would hold me likewise. I think the words I speak in this book are words I have accumulated within me for many years, and this is the year I have long awaited, an opportunity to share my dedication to scholarship and to writing.

12 Pyramid Stairs to Writing Analysis and Research

(See Appendix 1 for Pyramid Graphic)

The following steps are what I have created for effective analytic writing classes, and are a blend of some techniques I have learned and used in my writing and about the teaching of writing over decades of professional activities. I can assure CIA that I am not divulging any sacred methods because my research techniques are what I have personally developed over decades. This is a suggested methodology for teaching the research and analytic process:

Selecting and Evaluating Sources

Stair 1

Selecting and evaluating sources is critical to reading intelligence and open source material; both Top Secret and Open Sources are looked at with hawk's critical eye, and reliable sourcing must be tested and proven for authenticity, political bias, or any other thing that could influence or skew analysis of data. Analysts should also consider any political *deception* behind information that taints the reliability of the source. The study of source deception activates analyzing *perceptions management,* which can include deceptive statements by leaders, surreptitious placement of articles in newspapers, propaganda front groups, and the media as propaganda arms of governments. Student analysts must learn to discern that what they read from some media sources might be deliberately planted to deceive them (see Appendix 8 for source evaluation form). Young student analysts can begin to establish source legitimacy by answering:

- Who or what was the source?

- What is the source's access to the information? How did the source get the data?

- What is the source's creditability? Is the source distinguished, renown? Former information accurate?

- Does the information make sense?

 CIA analysts push through thousands of pages of research every week and remember *like connections*. These *connections* are the pyramidal base of a writer's analytic *first stair.* I encourage my students to seek out human sources within the university's varied departments, who will provide them with useful information on varied topics through a *formal interview* (see Appendix 9) for international writing topics). I also encourage my students to use unclassified IMINT (imagery intelligence) when researching topics like North Korean nuclear sites or flooding in New Orleans.[1]

Evidence for research derives from diverse sources, and inherent in each source are potential or actual *biases.* Evaluate the *reliability of sources* and begin to read a diverse array of material, then begin to make connections between and among people's names, associations, political affiliations, religious proclivities, economic trade connections, regional allies and whatever other host of *source testing questions* that you can come up with:

- Can you trust a Palestinian news source to say anything good about Israel or an Israeli source to say the same?

- Will Pakistan provide accurate information about India, and will India do the same?

- Why haven't we eliminated the poppy fields in Afghanistan?

- China not a threat to us?

- Why is the FBI still searching for Jimmy Hoffa's body in 2006?

- D' ya' think UBL might be in eastern Afghanistan or western Pakistan?

I like to think how I can analyze these queries, and establish *patterns of reliability* before selecting the sources I will use. I like to ask the question: what do the facts I have selected *indicate* on a larger level about my basic topic? These *indicators* will begin to germinate ideas and feed my analysis.

This procedure, of course, can easily be translated into the university classroom; this prepares graduates for future specialization in the arts and philosophies, engineering, computers, law, medical etc., and gives the ability to join the global economic community, while serving our great nation. I am not suggesting that we focus entirely on international political, religious or business topics, but that we engage writing about and remembering all the images and symbols and teachings we all bring to a large global table, which includes literature and the arts. Poets and actors are greatly valued in my long memory.

---

1   Unclassified IMINT data is easily accessed via INTERNET sources. Also, go to www.fas.org, Federation of American Scientists' (FAS) website for IMINT sources.

12 Pyramid Stairs to Research and Analysis

From *Writers Crossing Boundaries*

Stair 1: Source Evaluation

Stair 1. Selecting / evaluating sources critical to reading open source material:

- **should be looked at with hawk's critical eye.**

Sourcing must be tested/ proven for reliability:
- **authenticity**
- **political bias**
- **anything that influences/ skews analysis of data.**

Stair 1. Source Evaluation

Deception

- Media sources might be planted to deceive:

    –taints source reliability.

Perceptions management can include:

- deceptive statements by leaders.

- articles.

- propaganda front groups in media.

Stair 1. Source Evaluation

Student-analysts establish *Source Legitimacy* **by answering:**

1. Who/ what was the source?
2. What is source's access to information?
3. How did source get data?
4. What is source's credibility? Is source distinguished, renown? Former information accurate?
5. Does information make sense?
6. Is info verified by other sources?

Stair 1. **Source Evaluation**

Pyramidal Base – Memory
- Teach students to remember *like connections*.

Memory Connections:
- not just aptitude to recall facts, but to *recall patterns that relate factors to broader concepts.*

Stair 1. Source Evaluation

Begin to read diverse array of material, then make connections among:

- people's names
- associations: political affiliations
- religious proclivities
- economic trade connections
- regional allies
- whatever host of *source testing questions* you can come up with.

Stair 1. Source Evaluation

Use IMINT

- Encourage students to use unclassified IMINT (imagery intelligence).

- Research topics like North Korean nuclear sites or flooding in New Orleans[1]

(see Appendix 9 for international writing topics).

[1] Unclassified IMINT data is easily accessed via INTERNET sources. Also, **go to www.fas.org, Federation of American Scientists' (FAS)** website for IMINT sources.

Stair 1. Source Evaluation

Cognitive processing of info difficult:
- Encourage writer/analysts to *delineate assumptions and chains of inference.*
- *Particularize degree and source of* uncertainty involved in conclusions.
- Has evidence been consistent?

Writer/analysts create an analytic "reality" via sensory Input that is mediated by processes:
- *selection and disposal*
- *organizational clustering*
- *designation of meanings.*

Stair 1. Source Evaluation

Identifying Biases in diverse sources:

- Inherent in each source—potential or actual *biases.*

- Essential that analysts dispose of innate/ learned prejudices—*reactive mind* influences *reason*.

Stair 1: Source Evaluation

Gather data from contradictory sources:

- Information collected early stimulates writers to form tentative thesis, but *blurs importance of contradictory viewpoints.*

- ***Established perceptions*** often difficult to alter—thesis must be fluid.

ESTABLISHED PERCEPTIONS

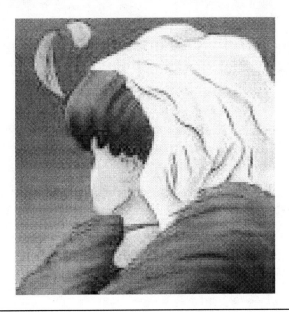

Stair 1. Source Evaluation

Human cognitive lenses disrupted by:

- mind-sets
- mental archetypes (symbols, images)
- prejudices
- analytic assumptions
- educational and cultural baggage.

Stair 1. Source Evaluation

Biases are disruptive to analytic processing:
- People construct *simplified models of reality* not applicable to complex problems.

    - *Motivational biases* come from ambitions and fears influencing our judgment.

    - *Cultural biases* predispose judgments in line with our heritage.

    - *Perceptual biases* construct rather than record "reality;" impedes accuracy of perceptions.

Stair 1. Source Evaluation

Cognitive biases influence:
- how an analyst estimates probabilities,

- evaluates evidence,

- attributes causality (Heuer 31-32)[1].

[1] See Heuer's article "Cognitive Factors in Deception and Counterdeception." <u>Strategic Miltary Deception.</u> Pergamon Press, 1982.

Stair 1. Source Evaluation

- Is there an imbalance in thought, emotion, or facts that makes the writer discount such information?

- Is the analytic writer in control of her biases that may skew *data disposal*?

- Didn't *Bakhtin* say I could ignore whatever voices I wanted?

Stair 1. Source Evaluation

Clustering : directed exercise in *Divergent/ Convergent* thinking (see Appendix 10):

- Divide into Teams; develop *data and source clusters* on information already known.
- Must be presented with a problem to solve.
- What are *logical connections* between what *evidence* the writer analyst gathered, and what information is *disposed of* either because it doesn't make sense or derives from a *biased* source?

Alternative Hypothesis

When analyzing any issue, the analyst should select from alternative hypotheses by asking:

- Which of several explanations is correct?
- Which of several outcomes is most likely?

The analytic process should contain the following elements:
- Identify all possible hypotheses. Brainstorm with others who have different perspectives.
- List the evidence for and against all hypotheses – include what is "absent."
- Determine evidence to judge likelihood of hypotheses. Prepare hypothesis matrix (See Appendix 11 for instructions to construct matrix).
- Refine matrix. Reconsider hypotheses; add/delete evidence and arguments.
- Try to refute hypotheses rather than confirm them.
- Report conclusions.

Stair 1. Source Evaluation

Patterns begin to emerge:
- political affiliations
- religious or economic connections
- flurries of diplomatic activities
- any pattern of any kind.

Have students write about patterns in their own lives—will see how predictable are peoples' behavior patterns:
- Predictable patterns of evidence emerge from sources.

CONTACT INFORMATION

Dr. Deborah M. Coulter-Harris

UH 5130Q

Office Telephone:419-530-4416

Home:

Email: <u>drdcharris@aol.com</u>

<u>deborah.coulter-harris@utoledo.edu</u>

Conducting the Interview

Stair 2

Students at this stage are still gathering information, so I require them to seek out professionals on campus who have knowledge of their topic; my students spread out to *interview* engineering, psychology, literary, medical etc. professionals, who can answer their questions and shed light on their research subject matter. This serves a twofold purpose: students conduct a professional interview with well-thought out questions, and they familiarize themselves with the academic excitement of campus life. Students begin to make *personal connections* with others, and learn *who possesses what information* on campus.

Beginning Analysis

Stair 3

Analysis of information can be done quickly if students learn to *process and organize* vital information into *categories*. *Clustering* information into dates, names or any other categories for closer scrutiny is advised; students should plug the information directly into a computer and create broad headlines to identify the *clusters*. Literature students can cluster language and artistic movements in philosophical-political eras. Now the analyst must see *emerging patterns* that might be germane to the formation of a *general thesis statement*.

I do not encourage my students to begin to formulate any type of thesis until they have collected and analyzed the facts and formulated an *unbiased voice* and *point of view* that responds accurately to the information. It is essential that the analyst disposes of innate or learned prejudices and does not let a *reactive mind* influence *reason*. Remember—no thesis statement prior to the start of research because "you don't know what you've got 'til you've got it." It is important that students gather a diverse array of data from contradictory sources. Information collected early stimulates writers to form a tentative thesis and tends to blur the importance of contradictory viewpoints, much like the young woman/old woman example provided earlier; established perceptions are often difficult to alter.

Cognitive processing of information can be difficult; it is essential to encourage writer/analysts to *delineate assumptions* and *chains of inference*, while also particularizing the degree and source of the uncertainty involved in conclusions. Writer/analysts create an analytic "reality" via sensory input that is mediated by processes that involve *selection and disposal, organizational clustering*, and *designation of meanings.* Analysts need to understand that human cognitive lenses are disrupted by mind-sets, mental archetypes, prejudices, or analytic assumptions—all the educational and cultural baggage we bring to the writing table. Richard Heuer identifies several types of biases that can disrupt analytic processing:

- People construct *simplified models of reality* not applicable to complex problems.

- *Motivational biases* come from out ambitions and fears influencing our judgment.

- *Cultural biases* predispose judgments in line with our heritage

- *Perceptual biases* construct rather than record "reality;" this impedes accuracy of perceptions.

- *Cognitive biases* influence how an analyst estimates probabilities, evaluates evidence, and attributes causality (Heuer 31-32).[2]

Directing Analysis

Stair 4

A good technique used to cluster information is an exercise in *Divergent/Convergent* thinking (see Appendix 10)[3]; divide the classroom into Teams and let them develop *data and source clusters* based on information they already know about the world. Students must be presented with a problem to solve:

---

2   See Heuer's article "Cognitive Factors in Deception and Counterdeception." <u>Strategic Miltary Deception.</u> Pergamon Press, 1982.

3   This technique was created by former CIA analyst, Morgan Jones in <u>The Thnker's Toolkit: 14 Powerful Techniques for Problem Solving,</u> New York: Times Business: Random House, 1998.

What are the *logical connections* between what *evidence* the writer analyst gathered, and what information is *disposed of* either because it doesn't make sense or derives from a *biased* source? Is there an imbalance in thought, emotion, or facts that makes the writer discount such information? Is the analytic writer in control of her biases that may skew *data disposal*? Didn't *Bakhtin*[4] say I could ignore whatever voices I wanted?

It is essential that *analysis* be directed away from political, class, gender, race, sexual biases, for that will slant the analysis in favor of personal beliefs. This might fly against decades old theories that encouraged writers to embrace their personal differences; this is a useful analytic technique in creative and more artistic writing classes, but university demographics prove the majority of students need professional and business writing skills that require unbiased analysis. Analysis is not about "the me"; a good analyst must be an impartial judge of accurate information and not be swayed by *cultural constructions*. So I see our writing departments expanding in analytic professional writing (see Appendix 11 for a sample of political analysis in the early stages of writing a report).

Analysts must also shy away from *group think*, and be able to present their ideas without fear of political repercussion in the classroom. Young analysts can cave to peer pressure about any number of beliefs, so they need to be reassured that individuality of thought is encouraged and embraced. The best analysts are able to process writing with haste, but remain accurate in weighing indicators of future events that could ultimately change their thesis. For example, you may plan to go to war, but if you have no plans to return home, then I think expanding influence and presence in the Middle East and Central Asia will eventually be a good thing for U.S. stability and security.

Formulating Thesis

Stair 5

There is any number of skills that should be taught to our writing students. After my students have completed the first four pyramidal stairs they are ready to begin to form their *point of view* towards the data and begin to think about writing a short, general analytic *thesis* statement. If students are writing an argument paper then the thesis statement must provide the *solution to the problem or controversy*, and they must provide a *refutation* in their paper that defines *the opposition* and generally destroys its position using *logic*. If some student papers are writing straight research without controversy they, of course, begin to form original ideas based on *data mining* and clustering.

---

4   I studied the Russian, literary theorist, M. M. Bakhtin, in graduate school.

Strategies for developing and evaluating thesis include *situational logic, application of theory,* and *comparison* (Heuer 32-38). Generating thesis with *situational logic* starts with concrete elements of unique conditions, and focuses on cause-effect or means-ends relationships (see Appendix 12 for a decision logic tree). For example, why would Al Qaeda operatives believe terrorist acts against America will achieve worldwide Islamic unity? Theories are generalizations based upon the study of many examples of some event or circumstance—when certain conditions arise, other conditions follow with certainty or some degree of probability. For example, the United States is attempting to make Iraq a democracy; this implies conditions that suggest conclusions about the military, security, and political process in Iraq. Based upon historical examples, will the United States be successful in attaining its goals? Can you define our goals for the next five years in the Middle East? This leads us to historical *analogic precedents* that can be used to fill gaps in understanding current conditions; the outcome of the present situation will likely be similar to the past, or a policy must be developed to avoid past outcomes based upon similar situations. *general to specific*   *specific to general*

Students need training in *deductive* and *inductive* thinking skills; most students from public urban schools have never been taught these mental exercises. Most of my classes produce a one-page essay every week using reasoning skills; this technique translates well into their longer argument and research papers. I encourage students to begin to focus on a topic of concern that relates to the local, national, and international community[5]—some problem that affects many at all levels. I encourage Team writing for at least one major project; working with others is a difficult skill to master, but is a requirement for success.

Portfolios

I usually ask students at this stage to begin to assemble an orderly portfolio of their research in the form of a large binder. The portfolio usually includes:

- All sources used with exclusion of books.

- All drafts: it's usually good to save versions of drafts in separate computer files in case you have to refer to some earlier information that you had deleted and now need.

---

5   Global issues are specified thematic angles— writing instructors can employ many topics and themes.

Writing Summaries

Stair 6

Writing analysis requires brevity of language and a rational voice; an analyst must be able to express ideas succinctly and strive to eliminate unnecessary words that add nothing to the meaning of what is being said, editing down adjectives and adverbs and unnecessary phrases. They must answer the question: What do the facts indicate? As government, the military, and the corporate world all use this type of writing, university students currently need these skills for future economic survival. You cannot enter these worlds and not know how to write a memorandum, quarterly analysis of projected profits and losses, or be able to accumulate data and analyze any number of types of impacts on US.

Students now write a *summary* of all their sources. Articles are summarized into very short paragraphs of four or five sentences that can later be edited down for *brevity*. They must also insert the appropriate *parenthetical citation* for the source at the end of this paragraph, which gives them a jump-start on tracking sources and beginning a temporary *Works Cited page*.[6] I advise students to only select chapters from books directly related to their topic—they need to quickly gather information and *begin to process;* the human mind is the greatest computer ever invented, but it needs training in *processing.*

Writing good summaries is an essential skill for research papers, as this concise information will be used as evidence to support unbiased, original analysis. Summaries are also useful:

- In clustering *like evidence*

- In data *disposal*

- At the first stages of analysis.

Writing Analytic Headers

Stair 7

Having organized the information into like paragraphs, analysts begin organizing and writing *short analytic Major and Minor Headers*[7] above paragraph sections; this easily sifts analysis and facts into logical sections, which is extremely useful for research writing. The headers also teach students that every paragraph must begin with an analytic statement followed by facts that support that analysis. Many new university writers think that just compiling facts makes a research paper; insisting on *analytic topic sentences* enables students to deeper understand what their *discovered clusters of indicators* are saying.

---

6   Students should learn to access MLA (Modern Language Association) Internet source examples.

7   **MAJOR** headers should be all caps and bolded and should be doubled spaced above paragraphs; **Minor Headers** should use lower case and appear bolded directly above paragraph sections.

When analyzing any issue, the analyst should select from alternative hypotheses by asking:

- Which of several explanations is correct?

- Which of several outcomes is most likely?

The analytic process should contain the following elements:

- Identify all possible hypotheses. Brainstorm with others who have different perspectives.

- List the evidence for and against all hypotheses – include what is "absent."

- Determine evidence to judge likelihood of hypotheses. Prepare hypothesis matrix (See Appendix 11 for instructions to construct matrix).

- Refine matrix. Reconsider hypotheses; add/delete evidence and arguments.

- Try to refute hypotheses rather than confirm them.

- Report conclusions.

Writing the Synthesis

Stair 8

Writing synthesis is the most fun because *patterns* begin to emerge. These patterns can be any number of items: political affiliations, religious or economic connections, flurries of diplomatic activities that can be monitored on the Internet, that lets you know who's visiting whom on what date and where—or, any other type of pattern. If a cow goes into a field to eat periodically, you can pretty much rely on that cow to be there at some point in the future.

Have students write about the patterns in their own lives in a short essay, and they will see how predictable are the patterns of peoples' behaviors. This exercise makes them aware of how predictable patterns of evidence emerge from sources, and how easy it is to glean truth from falsehood. Students should have already scrutinized and disposed of biased evidence, so they no longer subscribe to every notion they read as ultimate truth; they need to distinguish between propaganda and fact.

Writing synthesis is an exercise in organizing by *theme.* Students can begin to synthesize their analyses and test opposing theories; they can then begin to formulate a *rough thesis statement.* At this stage student analysts should have already tested the reliability of their sources, and disposed of information that no longer supports the analysis. The synthesis stair is primary in organizing paragraph placement, and in constructing a solid first draft.[8]

Integrating Graphics

Stair 9

Integration of graphics with photos, charts, tables, etc. must be carefully selected to enhance the analysis; student analysts should be discouraged from *plopping* in graphics that are irrelevant to supporting the thesis. Labeling and writing *captions* for graphics is another requirement for professional writing. I also require a graphic cover page—this encourages creativity. Although not all research writing requires a graphic element, I think allowing students to connect *visual signs* that strengthen and enhance the meaning of their papers is exciting for me to read as an instructor. I am usually overwhelmed at the outcome.

I usually instruct my students not to "reinvent the wheel," as they are likely to find graphics on the Internet that will correspond to their analysis. Key to this stair is understanding that graphic sources must be listed on the *Works Cited* page, and that *graphic insertion does not mushroom* in the paper and overcome the text. Three to five graphics is all that should be required of a ten-page research paper.

Parenthetical citations are also required to source graphic material and should be located at the end of the caption. I encourage students to include *NOTES* and *Appendices* in their papers, so they learn the value of what information is vital to the main paper and what information is supplemental in importance. Students enjoy creating complex charts—most have sophisticated computer skills already.

Forecasting

Stair 10

An *Outlook and Future Indications* section at the end of research papers are encouraged, by formulating such questions as:

---

8   For experienced writers and thinkers, the synthesis stage can occur concurrently during a
     polished draft.

- What do you see in the future regarding this problem or controversy?

- How will your assessment affect our nation's community for good or ill?

- What do you see happening in the near or the distant future regarding your topic?

- How will this affect the local, national, or international community?

- Why should we care?

(See Appendix 13 for a sample chart evaluation of a research project).

Coordination with others

Stair 11

Student analysts must now seek out at least two experts in their research topic fields, and *coordinate* with a student colleague. Students should rely on the sound advice of others to test the future success of the research paper. This is a slightly more expansive method than *peer review* because it invites others outside the classroom to participate in student projects.

Briefing[9]

Capstone 12

Briefings are an integral part of analytic writing, and the capstone to a student's personal achievement. After gaining expertise in a *focused area of information* or *account*, the students are ready to give *briefings*. I like to conduct informal briefings and collaborative conversation with students about their projects. They need to learn to respond to *interrupting questions* or comments during briefings—real world writing isn't as polite as academia. Students learn to defend their position through logic and sound analysis of data; students must extract a one-page outline from their papers, and present their *Key Findings* to their peers. I usually allow for a ten to fifteen minute question and answer period following the briefing; this technique strengthens students' ability to "think on their feet." This exercise is also a vehicle to develop a writer's *voice*.

Briefings are the oral culmination of research and writing, and students do not have to stand. Students should appear comfortable enough to talk about their *area of expertise*; if any student panics from shyness, let them remain silent;

---

9   No one writing outside the Academy uses the term "oral presentations."

I never force anyone to brief.[10] Briefings should be ten to 15 minutes and slightly longer for Team briefings, which are followed by the question period. All students are required to write at least one thoughtful question during the briefing, which leads to enlivened discussions.

---

10   I have found that only one or two students in a year will not volunteer to brief.

Creative Writing Experience

Growth in Artistic Writing

I was schooled in Latin for twelve years and my mother spoke French, so my ability to write and understand other languages had been enhanced with environment, classical training, and the study of classical logic and argument[1]; argument demands an understanding of structures and rules and order, which are essential for analytic writing. I began writing poetry when I was twelve years old largely because my Irish grandmother Margaret [nee Corley] Coulter gave me a copy of Frost's enthralling *In the Clearing*. There should be excitement at varied types of readings and a very large catalogue of writing courses in our universities that are not necessarily textbook driven; narrow writing theories and old political ideologies are not apropos in a global reorder.

My favorite venue to write through is creative writing; I like using the readers' mind like canvas and paint images that connect to events. I like playing with sounds using words as bells or trumpets; I enjoy wondering what my images will conjure in my readers' heads, and whether or not anyone will really understand the message. I'm learned to pare down words now in my poetry.

I began life as a poet and my poetic writing skills were tested in Dublin, Ireland, many years ago. I knew all the famous Irish poets, and I used to read with them in public readings (to see examples of my published poetry, please refer to Appendix 14); most of these poets are still alive: Leland Bardwell, Ulick O'Connor, Macdara Woods, Pearse Hutchinson, Eilean Ni Chuilleanain—I knew them all. I met the widow Katherine Kavanagh in Boston and Dublin.[2] I had a cottage on the Irish Sea near Beatrice Behan,[3] and spent time on Lambay Island at a castle during August harvest with Lord Rupert Revelstoke of Bearing Banks fame; I liked to lobster fish during summer and sail the Irish Sea (see Appendix 15 for a poem on that experience).

During my travels abroad, I met Holocaust survivors in England; their names were Ilsa and Elsa, twins. One of the twins was a hunchbacked dwarf, and the other sister married an Oxford Don. They told me of the night they were arrested and taken to a Concentration Camp in Germany. Ilsa jumped several floors to the street and ruined her hearing and was arrested by the Gestapo; Elsa made escaped to

---

1   The nuns taught us syllogisms in Catholic elementary school.
2   Katherine was the widow of the late Irish poet Patrick Kavanagh.
3   Beatrice Behan is the widow of Brendan Behan.

England, and she and the Don paid for Ilsa's release just before the slaughter. These sisters took me to visit Cambridge and the glorious city of Bath.

There was a magical Irish actress, Maureen A'Hearn, who groomed me in Dublin for the stage; I appeared on many stages in Ireland when young. I met Maureen after being cast in the show, *Masters and Servants*, which was an adaptation of Jonathan Swift. She wore a gold fox hat and lived in people's attics. Our company toured universities and stately homes in Northern Ireland. I remember calling my father back in Massachusetts to let him know I was in Belfast—he was quite shocked. Maureen's father was the famous Irish actor, Brian A'Hearn, and her mother came from British royalty. She was quite elegant and dramatic and exceptionally well-groomed. Unfortunately, Maureen followed her mother's earlier example and committed suicide in the 1980s and was buried in a potter's field.

I studied acting at the Abbey Theatre with Patrick Mason, who later became the Artistic Director of the Abbey—I never missed a single class. Patrick was a great vocal and movement teacher. I studied under Christopher Casson[4] and Dr. Hilton Edwards at the Gate Theatre; this theatre trained in the classical style of British acting and taught me to project my voice without microphones. Some guys at CIA mistakenly thought I talked loudly because I came from New England, but my volume generally increases when confronted with a crowd. Mr. Casson was successful in teaching me how to pronounce "Duke" properly; he continually reminded me that I was not introducing John Wayne—"d'yuke", Deborah, "d'yuke—say d'yuke," he would say.

A challenging task in Dublin was writing and performing my own radio show, "Poet's Choice," at RTE Radio on Saturday nights. I read my poetry and the writing of others and sang American Revolutionary War songs and old English and Irish ballads. RTE recorded well over an hour of my singing after my radio show was over, but the tape disappeared and I never got to hear what I sounded like then. I also performed in many plays in Ireland, and was fortunate to have shared the stage three times with the famous Irish actor, Gabriel Byrne.

Although my professional life has interrupted my artistic writing, for the first time in years I was able to return to my roots in poetry during summer 2005, and wrote a verse play, *The Hanging Gardens of Babylon,* my first verse play; the play's Forward is included at the end of this essay (see Appendix 16). I wanted to include a piece of new academic work in the Introduction to the Opera that relates to my varied interests in religion, antediluvian history, literature, and archaeology— to what had interested me of late; I also wanted to include my most recent artistic piece for review. My love for language and writing began with immersion in literature—I favor early Neoclassical British Literature and Irish and American

---

4   Christopher Casson was the son of Dame Sybil Thorndike; he was a renown actor on stage and film.

poetry. I like to chant in Latin and Hebrew. Words were the primary part of my literacy training from youth in private Catholic schools; students then could recite long poems from memory and speak Mass by memory in Latin, useful training *techniques in memory and language.*

Literary analysis requires the same demands as professional writing, but is more introspective into character, word choices, etc. I was trained in literary analysis, which served me very well at CIA; literary and intelligence analyses are not that divergent in finding *patterns and formulas.* I also like to write satire, for I enjoyed studying Swift and actually played satirist Dean Swift in a theatrical tour I did in Northern Ireland. I wrote of number of political satires while living in Philadelphia (see Appendix 17). Studying linguistics is a requirement for the development of analysts, helping them to distinguish patterns in language and customs. I like to study the origins of language, and get to the root of the word. I am fascinated to study how words deceive, how words are used in propaganda, and it is up to the analyst to make that "deception" call. An analyst must always remember to question the *intent* and *source reliability* of the manuscript, and pay honor to "doubt." Encourage writers to consider doubts by listing *information gaps* that are obstacles to sound judgment.

Interest in Religion

I hope the reader will indulge me briefly on the last section of this letter before the Outlook, and allow me to write a few thoughts on religious conflicts. Much of my life has involved the study of religion; I am interested in current religious conflicts and how they are being played out on the global political stage. I think Samuel Huntington was correct predicting in 1993, in his original essay "The Clash of Civilizations,"[5] that future wars would be the product of religious and cultural divides. Anti-secular movements' — in the Middle East, Africa, Southeast Asia, Asia and the Islands — intent is to build a unified wall that embraces Europe and the Americas as well. Religious turmoil between Muslims and others in Great Britain and France already sparks endless violence and duplicity. The renewal and rise of Messianic traditions—which are "full of shared visions of social breakdown, climatic disaster, wars and rumors of wars as precursors to the appearance of the Savior" (Hogue 17)—increase the risk of global religious fractures.

In July, 2006, we saw a new conflict developing between Hezbollah and Israel. This would be a convenient time to bring on Armageddon with chilled relations between Russia and the United States and with Asia ready to pounce on us. The fact that so many illegals have entered our country and our government's delay in rescuing 25, 000 Americans from Lebanon and the poor response time to New Orleans, should be a wake-up call to US citizens that your government cannot fully protect you. As one of the chief mandates to government leaders is the security contract they have with their citizens, we need to expand our military, and the US Army should have a minimum of 2.5 million active duty. WE might want to consider drafting the illegals for our infantry. If they want to become US citizens, then let them serve their country like my grandfathers did, one in Cuba during the Spanish American War, and one in World War I.

Building Global Religious Walls

Religion is the organizing principle of Middle Eastern, Asian, and African societies; I would like to question whether United States' foreign policy planning includes methodologies—other than war— to weaken anti-secular, theocratic ideologies that destabilize regions and threaten U.S. security? As political lines are being increasingly drawn in the international community upon religious boundaries, it may be best to agree with Robert Frost that, "Good fences make good neighbors," that it's not so much what you're walling in – but what you are walling out. Maybe the western territory of Iraq could be a partial solution to the Israeli-Palestinian problems with water and land; both Israelis and Palestinians could expand their

---

5   I am not including the text of this article in my book as it is easily accessed on the Internet

territories east and could receive water from the Tigris and Euphrates. After all, Israel has been trying to organize water deliveries from Turkey for a least a decade.[6]

Religious Divisions Strengthen Nationalism

A profession of ethnic- national identity often involves religious intolerance and discrimination against those not identified. There are many "messianic" and "chosen" religions that connect directly with race or ethnicity and many are within national borders. According to David Little from the *United States Institute of Peace* (USIP), "Religious ideas are often associated with ethnicity and nationalism: a 'chosen people' with a divine mission," as well as a belief in the superiority of cultural values, and, "… the right to form an "autonomous polity in the name of advancing a holy mission. Hebrew Scripture, whether interpreted by Jews or Christians, the Qur'an, and some significant Buddhists doctrines and texts, for example, all provide the foundation and the inspiration for enlisting political and military power in the cause of defending and advancing certain sacred values and ways of life" (Little 1995).

Religious global trends indicate more religious *fracture zones* occurring via these "autonomous polities," but the novel idea is that of global and political domination by a singular religion and its call to submission. Nationalists often favor a repressive ideology, which demands strict adherence to a national tradition that includes the dominant religion, which compels and controls both religious belief and political behavior. Sometimes, I wonder if a person's religion is simply an accident of geographic birth and inheritance, or if our Heavenly Father laughs at all our religious nonsense? It appears some religions have one predominate race or tribe of people attached; this begs the question whether ancient local gods were transformed into hyperbolic Nationalist gods.

Islam and Judaism

Presently, the Islamic world in the Middle East and North Africa is enveloped by a resurgent Islamic fundamentalism, partially as a response of the inequities of globalization. Islamic fundamentalist insurgencies, funded by rogue states and terrorist organizations, are trying to destabilize the moderate, Western-leaning, secular regimes currently in power, and are seeking to replace them with a unified, resuscitated Islamic Caliphate (empire). According to a National Intelligence Council (NIC) report, "Religion, and specifically Islam, has increasingly become the prime identifier in recent years. Whether it continues in that role or not, the question of identity will be a major influence on regional events. A continued emphasis on Islam as an identifying attribute would color regional politics, define

---

6   One of the last Turkish plans was to deliver water to Israel in giant bladders.

possible major regime changes, set limits on economic and social policies, and help define relations with outside powers" (NIC 2003)[7].

Genesis of Arab-Israeli Conflict

Some might argue the Arab-Israeli Wars of the last 55 years, and the subsequent unstable situation have not been religious-based, but it appears the genesis of these conflicts was. According to the Old Testament, included in the *Torah*, the conflict began between *Isaac* and *Ishmael*, the latter being the son of Abraham's concubine, but his first born son. Ishmael would not inherit the Throne of the kingdom of Israel because it belonged to Abraham's first legitimate son, Isaac, with his wife, *Sarah*. Succeeding generations of these sides, therefore, have continued in this ancient tribal feud.

History reveals that hostility in the Middle East has participated in an overemphasis of religious differences among Islam and Judaism and Christianity. The re-creation of a State of Israel in May 1948 recalled - for the first time in centuries - their conflict almost exclusively in the Middle East. Costs have been expensive for all sides. After the 1948 War, more than 700,000 Jews in 8 Arab countries fled for their lives, their property ransacked, and their schools, hospitals, synagogues and cemeteries expropriated or destroyed. On the other hand, hundreds of thousands of Palestinians were either forced from their lands after the UN founding of the state of Israel, or tragically, have remained quarantined in squalid camps meagerly sustained by UN and Arab countries' aid. These camps are hotbeds of anarchy.

Genesis of Arab-Israeli Conflict

Some might argue the Arab-Israeli Wars of the last 55 years, and the subsequent unstable situation have not been religious-based, but it appears the genesis of these conflicts was. According to the Old Testament, included in the *Torah*, the conflict began between *Isaac* and *Ishmael*, the latter being the son of Abraham's concubine, but his first born son. Ishmael would not inherit the Throne of the kingdom of Israel because it belonged to Abraham's first legitimate son, Isaac, with his wife, *Sarah*. Succeeding generations of these sides, therefore, have continued in this ancient tribal feud.

Religion is the festering wound of Middle East tensions. While Israel—waiting for Messiah to come — supports a quasi-democratic government, the reality of Israeli nationalist politics is centered on the Jewish belief that the nation of Israel derives its validity from religious prophecy – that it is the "restored nation" entitled to settle in the old "Promised Land." Muslims, by contrast, want to remove all traces of the

---

7   This unclassified CIA publication is easily accessible by visiting www.cia.gov

Jewish population in Israel and plan to make Jerusalem (Al Qods) the capital of the Islamic World Caliphate. Christians—waiting for Lord Jesus and His angels— demand a stake in the territory because of their belief in His return, who is thought —by both Jews and Arabs—to have been a prophet, but not the Son of God.

Rise of a Shiite Political Bloc in Iraq

Iraq is now the central force driving events in the Middle East. The outcome of the religious-based guerrilla insurgency, the U.S. occupation, and the shape of the future Iraqi government will impact the entire region and create other religious and cultural alliances. The emergence of the Shiite sect in Iraq as the dominant power in government makes Iraq the only Shiite-controlled Arab state.[1] Iraq's Iranian Shiite neighbors are delighted by the rise of the Iraqi Shia: Will Iran successfully export Shiite religious identity into Baghdad to supersede an Iraqi nationalist agenda? Stabilizing Iraq as a secular democratic state would give Washington unprecedented leverage in its relations with Middle Eastern states, but an anti-democratic religious-based Shiite regime friendly with Iran would create a powerful fundamentalist bloc that presages more religious-political turmoil for the next several decades. It is important that we stabilize Iraq.

Future Religious-Political Implications

During the Cold War, little attention was paid religious studies, as nation-builders evaluated religious-political conjunctions as marginal. "In Western political systems an absolute line had been drawn between man's spiritual life and his public actions, between religion and politics. The West de-secularized politics and de-politicized religion; western opinion viewed religion as irrational and pre-modern; a throwback to the dark centuries before the Enlightenment taught the virtues of rationality and decency, and bent human energies to constructive, rather than destructive purposes" (Weigel, 1991: 27). Secularization of the Middle East must still be considered essential for progress.

Future 'new wars' will end being patterned on classic interstate war. *Religious agents* have carried out recent terrorist violence; although, religiously aligned states could play a supporting role. "Such wars will not typically be triggered by a state interest, but by religious identity, zeal and fanaticism. The goal is not territory, as in "'old wars', but, "… to gain political power through generating fear and hatred. War then is political mobilization in which the pursuit of violence promotes extremist religious causes" (Held 2001).

Notes

1   Iran, controlled by a Shiite Theocracy, is not an Arab but a Persian state.

2   The Jewish/Islamic conflict is not limited to the Middle East. In late December 2000, two Islamic men stopped a school bus carrying 50 Jewish children between the ages of 8 and 10 at gunpoint near Paris, France, and residents of the mainly Arab suburb stoned the vehicle. It was believed that the incident was related to some 200 attacks against Jews or Jewish property by Muslims in France earlier that year in October. In fact, according to a French government report issued in early 2002, acts of violence against the Jews increased from one in 1998 to nine in 1999 to 116 in 2000. If one includes other anti-Semitic incidents, ranging from threats to arson, the numbers went from 74 in 1998 to 603 in 2000. In early 2002, the conflict between the Jews and Muslims outside of the Middle East took a new turn for the worst. On March 30th 15 young masked Muslim immigrants in Lyons, France rammed stolen cars through a Jewish synagogue's front gate, crashing into the temple's front doors. It was one of more than 300 anti-Jewish incidents in France, home to 6 million Muslims, in a 3-week period, compared with 200 in all of 2001. Sharp increases in attacks on Jews were reported in Britain, Russia and Belgium as well. Some called this a new wave of anti-Semitism in Europe (Religious Tolerance.org 2004).

Outlook:

Final Thoughts on Global Issues

The value of University is discourse and collegial discussion of a multitude of ideas; I believe narrow ideas crept into academic programs that could not keep pace with times. Some theories had value, but I think writing courses addressing a variety of global issues—religion, politics, terrorism, global warming and the such—will better prepare students to meet current global demands. Business and Professional Writing Programs need to be strengthened to address the needs of the majority of computer, engineering, medical etc. students, and this type of professional writing requires structure, form, and logic. All students should have the opportunity to select a writing course that will meet the larger needs of their collective future. Logic must be central to curriculum. I think the *era of introspection* is over, and an *era of analysis and remembering* has begun—*writing for the real world*, writing for real.

Sincerely thanks,
Deborah,
20 June, 2006

Images From Summer 2006

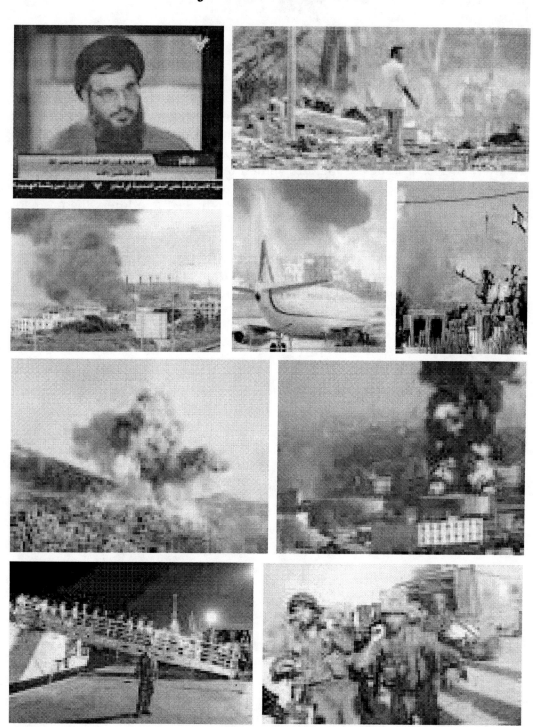

Map of the Middle East

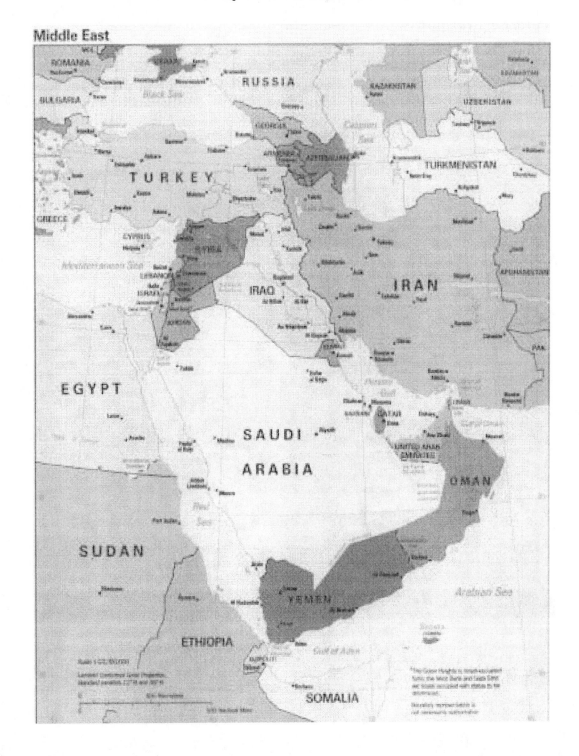

Appendix 1

Pyramid Graphic

12 Pyramid Stairs to Research and Analysis

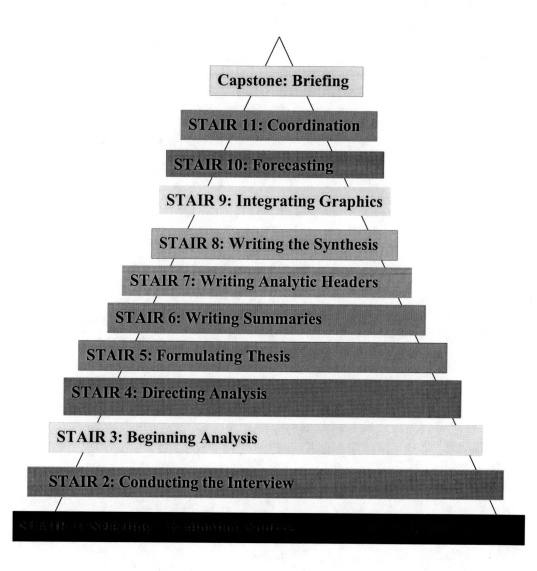

Capstone: Briefing

STAIR 11: Coordination

STAIR 10: Forecasting

STAIR 9: Integrating Graphics

STAIR 8: Writing the Synthesis

STAIR 7: Writing Analytic Headers

STAIR 6: Writing Summaries

STAIR 5: Formulating Thesis

STAIR 4: Directing Analysis

STAIR 3: Beginning Analysis

STAIR 2: Conducting the Interview

STAIR 1: Selecting, Obtaining Sources

Appendix 2a

Copy of request to review letter sent to CIA 2 June, 2006.

Dr. Deborah M. Coulter-Harris
XXXXXXXXXXXXXXXXXX
Toledo, Ohio XXXXX

1 June, 2006

Chairman,
Publication Review Board
1G03 IP Building
Washington, D.C. 20505

Dear Chairman:

I am including a copy of an essay I was asked to write this summer by a colleague at the University of Toledo; I am to submit an early draft within two weeks. My essay is entitled "Publishing in the Profession—Writing for Real." This essay may continue on as a book, and I will make sure you are given final drafts prior to submissions.

Thank you for your cooperation in this matter; I hope you enjoy the essay.

Sincerely yours,

Dr. Deborah M. Coulter-Harris

Appendix 2b

Copy of Request to review letter sent to CIA on 20 June, 2006.

Dr. Deborah Coulter-Harris
XXXXXXXXXXXXXX
Toledo, Ohio XXXXX
Tel. XXX-XXX-XXXX

20 June, 2006

Chairman
Publication Review Board
1G03 IP Building
Washington, D. C. 20505

Dear Chairman:

I am including the final 215 page draft of *Publishing in the Profession—Writing for Real*; I sent an earlier draft in the form of a 35 page essay on 1 June, 2006. As stated previously in my original letter about the project, I was asked to write this project by a colleague at the University of Toledo. Last summer, 2005, you approved my verse play, *The Hanging Gardens of Babylon*, which is included as Appendix 16 in the enclosed draft.

Thank you for your cooperation in this matter. I would appreciate hasty approval. Enjoy the book.

Sincerely yours,

Dr. Deborah M. Coulter-Harris,
Former CIA Analyst

Appendix 2c

CIA approval of this manuscript, received 1 July, 2006.

Subj:	PRB Approval
Date:	6/30/06 11:01:45 AM Eastern Daylight Time

From: kateem@ucia.gov (kateem)
To: drdcharris@aol.com, prb@ucia.gov (prb)

Dear Dr. Coulter-Harris:

The Publications Review Board has completed its review of your manuscript "Publishing in the Profession— Writing for Real." The Board has no objection to its publication. The Board appreciates your cooperation with prepublication review. This e-mail serves as the Board's official notification of review approval. If you wish, we can send you a signed letter to the same effect.

Please contact the Publications Review Board at 703-613-3070 if you have any questions or if we can be of further assistance.

Sincerely,

Kate/PRB Staff

Appendix 3

Web sources for study of religious conflict

http://www.academicinfo.net/Religionlibrary.html

http://www.adherents.com/

http://virtualreligion.net/vri/

http://www.sosig.ac.uk redirect?url=http%3A%2F%2 Fwww.skepsis.nl%2 Fonlinetexts. html&rec=10003750812800

http://www.sosig.ac.uk/roads/subject-listing/World-cat/socrel.html

http://agenda.religion.info/

http://aps.naples.net/community/NFNWebpages/storyboard.cfm?StoryBoardNum=142 &PageNum=40

http://www.incore.ulst.ac.uk/services/cds/themes/religion.html

http://www.cdr.dk/library_paper/lp-98-1.htm

http://www.osce.org/news/generate.php3?news_id=2800

http://www.wcrp.org/

http://www.fathom.com/feature/35583

http://www.adherents.com/Religions_By_Adherents.html

http://www.global-dialog.org/mvd/mvl.cgi?NextName=wWTC.religion.spirituality. html

http://www.etown.edu/vl/research.html

http://www.etown.edu/vl/research.html

http://www.bbc.co.uk/religion/news/indepth/review/

http://www.fpa.org/newsletter_info2583/newsletter_info.htm

http://www.quinnell.us/religion/links/info.html

http://www.workmall.com/wfb2001/lebanon lebanon_history religious_conflicts.html

http://www.columbia.edu/cu/lweb/indiv/africa/icrbib.html

http://csf.colorado.edu/peace/academic.html

http://agenda.religion.info/ndex.php?pageNum_Recordset1=4&totalRowsRecordset1=55

http://www.colorado.edu/conflict/bin/natdoc.cgi?keyword=cnflt_abs

http://www.hawaii.edu/powerkills/VIOLENCE.HTM

http://www.geostrategy-direct.com/geostrategy-direct/wnd.html

http://www.gwu.edu/~nsarchiv/

http://www.eppc.org/

http://www.state.gov/s/inr/

http://www.merip.org/

Appendix 4

Notes on classical thinkers

Topic: Contrast the education of the guardians in books ii and iii with the education of philosophers in book VII of *the republic.*

The Education of the Guardians

In Books II and III of *The Republic*, Socrates discusses various classes of people in a city, ending with the highest class, the rulers or guardians, who require the highest qualities. They must be courageous and philosophical, brave and wise. This leads to the subject of education, which, Socrates says, must consist of "gymnastic" for the body, and "music" for the soul. Plato believes that education begins in the nursery with fables and fairy stories, which he believes must be carefully censored to ensure a suitable moral tone; and, in particular, the gods must always appear in a virtuous light. Gods must be portrayed as the author of only good. They must never be portrayed as perpetrators of evil, or as capable of any falsehood.

In order to account for the preponderance of evil in the world, Plato has Socrates stating,"...the poets must find the kind of explanation we are seeking, and say that the actions of the gods are good and just, and that those who receive punishment are benefitted thereby...to say that the god, himself good, is the cause of evil for anyone, that we shall fight in every way, and we shall not allow anyone to say it in his own city."

- The tales of the battles between gods are not to be told to children, for students will be taught that it is disgraceful to quarrel with another citizen. The earliest lessons of education are to appeal to that element of virtue in the soul, elements that cause people to pursue the highest and most noble qualities of human nature.

" Music," in Plato's terms, applies to the education in literature, as well as in music proper. The term "gymnastic" applies to a whole system of diet and exercise, which would produce health and strength, a preparation for military service. In this system of education, Plato asserts that the soul, and not the body, is the primary object of "gymnastic" and "music." "Music" educates the philosophic part of the soul, while "gymnastic" disciplines the psychological element of the "spirit."

Plato also believes that the child, who is to be a soldier and to fight for his country, must learn not to be afraid of death. Plato wishes to banish the horrid pictures of Hades from poetry, and "...all those names of things in the underworld which make every hearer shudder." Plato believes that the Guardians should fear slavery more than death. Thus, according to Plato, if a man is not afraid to die himself, he will not be afraid for his friends to die, eliminating the need for "lamentations and pitiful speeches," which Plato considers unmanly. If grief is then a sign of weakness, its opposite emotion, laughter, must not be allowed as acceptable behavior. Plato considers that the violent expression of either feeling produces violent emotional reactions in people. Moderation in "...drink, sex, and food," will be taught as a virtue, as principles of balance and control, as important for the formation of character in childhood and early youth.

Plato emphasizes the manner or form of poetry, that is the *mode* in which the poet represents the characters in the poem: whether the poet speaks in his own person and simply describes or "narrates" what they say or do, or whether the poet should take on the persona of the character and "imitate" their speech and actions. Plato is actually dealing with the question of whether "imitation," or impersonation, should be the ruling principle in poetry, with the poet assuming the many personalities of his characters, or whether there might be some other criterion of poetic excellence, other than "imitative power."

Plato states that, "...when a moderate man in his narrative comes upon the words or actions of the good man he will be willing to expound it in character and not be ashamed of that kind of imitation...but he will do so much less when the good man is overcome by disease or sexual passion, or by drunkenness or some other misfortune...When he comes upon a character unworthy of himself, he will be unwilling to make himself seriously like that worse character." In this "imitative" capacity, Plato sees a danger to both the poet and his to the poet's audience. Plato is convinced that it is impossible for one man to excel in many trades and professions, so that it is impossible for one man (poet) to imitate many things very well.

- As for the "...man who in his cleverness can become many persons and imitate all things," Plato states that the city will "...bow down to him as being holy, wondrous," but he shall not be allowed to perform in this new city.

Plato states that musical songs, which are to be used in education, are composed of three elements: " words, musical mode and rhythm." The words must conform to the same rules of poetic topics already discussed. The "musical mode and rhythm" must be used to express those qualities which Plato deems appropriate in developing "...a truly good and fine character." Plato believes that artists and craftsman must be prevented from expressing what is "...vicious, mean, unrestrained or graceless." The young citizens of the new city are not to grow up amongst images of evil because their souls will assimilate the evil and ugliness of their surroundings.

Plato concludes *Book III* by stating that the object of the education of the Guardians is "...to attain the greatest degree of gentleness towards each other and toward those whom they are protecting."

The Education of Philosophers

Socrates begins *Book VII* with the story of the cave, which illustrates the escape of the philosophers from the fetters and darkness of the physical world of the senses, "...the realm of the visible," to the freedom and dazzling radiance of the world of the mind, "...the brightest of realities, which we say is the Good." However, Plato believes that the philosopher must afterwards return to the cave to enlighten and free those who are still imprisoned there.

The escape from the cave is made possible through the study of a number of subjects that deal with abstractions. Arithmetic, the study of "numbers and calculations," is seen as "...very necessary for a warrior to be able to count and calculate," and for the philosopher "...because he must emerge from the world of becoming and grasp reality, or never be a rational thinker."

Plane and solid geometry are to be studied, especially "...as it pertains to war... regarding encampments, occupations of positions, concentration and deployment of troops." Plato regards the study of calculations and geometry as being part of "...all things (that) tend in that direction which compel the soul to turn itself toward the place in which the most blessed part of reality exists, which the soul must see at any cost." Solid geometry is to be studied for developing perceptions of the third dimension, as in the study of cubes.

Astronomy is the third subject to be studied, as "...a better perception of the seasons and the months and years concerns not only the farmer and the navigator, but no less the general." Plato describes astronomy as being the study of the "...motion of things which have depth," in so far as it concerns the principle of movement of solids. Plato compares harmonics, the study of sound, to the study of astronomy. "The consonants and sounds, which they hear, they measure against each other and so labour in vain, as do the astronomers...as the eyes are fixed upon astronomy, so the ears are fixed upon the movements of harmony."

Plato believes that these studies have practical application, but their real value lies in their power to lead the soul out of veiled senses to the abstract world of the mind. Having been taught in abstract thinking, the Guardians will learn, through the study of dialectic, to understand the idea of what is "good." " So whenever a person tries through dialectic, and without any help from the senses, but by means of reason, to set out to find each true reality and does not give up before apprehending the Good itself with reason alone, that person reaches the final goal of the intelligible, just as the prisoner escaping the cave reached the final goal of the visible."

In the last part of **Book VII,** Plato describes the practical applications of his curriculum. After the standard education in music and gymnastic, the students pass on to the abstract subjects and then to dialectic, with frequent tests on the way. Those Guardians, from ages thirty five to fifty, " ...must be compelled to rule on matters of war and the government of youth, so that they shall not be inferior to others in experience." The few who reach the summit, who have survived all the tests, at the age of fifty, will divide their lives between philosophy and " public affairs."

CHAPTER 11. Aristotle's Poetics: *PARTS OF THE PLOT: REVERSAL, RECOGNITION, SUFFERING [Aristotle]*

Reversals and recognitions were introduced in **Chapter Ten** of *Aristotle's Poetics* as constructive elements, as differentiating ingredients within simple and complex plots. Simple imitative plots were those constructed of actions, during which changes in fortunes occurred, without the elements of reversals or recognitions. By contrast, Aristotle argued that complex plots had to include reversals and recognitions when a change in fortune appeared in the plot of the tragedy.

Aristotle defines reversals and recognitions as *changes* from a particular state to its opposite state, changes that must occur within a tragedy. Reversals and recognitions can then be considered as special categories of structural forms, which constitute tragic changes, or which influence the form the tragedy may take, when its plot is complex.

A reversal is a change of events or a change in the events of the tragic plot towards what is considered to be those particular events' opposites. In **Chapter Nine**, Aristotle had stated that "...incidents involving pity and fear are most effective when they come unexpectedly....things that actually do happen by accident seem most marvelous when they appear to be intentional." A reversal, then, is an unexpected but rational shift in the events in the play, such as from happiness to unhappiness or its reverse, and which includes a sudden reversal of fortune.

The whole reason for the sudden structural paradox in tragedy was explained, in **Chapter Nine**, as a dilemma which produced the desired emotional effects on the audience or the reader, the effects of pity or fear being "...most effective when they come unexpectedly."

At the beginning of **Chapter Eleven,** Aristotle attempts to give an example of reversal, but creates complications for the reader when he states that "...the messenger comes to cheer Oedipus by relieving him of fear with regard to his mother, but by revealing his true identity, does just the opposite of this." How could this messenger know about Oedipus' "fears," but until after he had arrived and spoken with Oedipus? Also, from Aristotle's statement, it is unclear whether it is the messenger or Oedipus himself who experiences the reversal.

- Recognition, the other structural form, tied to the complex tragedy, which accounts for changes in the plot's action, is the change from ignorance to knowledge. The rest of the definition of recognition in **Chapter Eleven** explains what makes the change tragic, and how this change corresponds to the pattern of tragic reversals.

In Chapter Fourteen, Aristotle analyzed the kind of injuries, which were considered to be tragic, " which seem terrible or pitiful." He indicated that there was nothing very tragic about an enemy injuring or killing his enemy, or about other characters injuring or killing one another when they were "...nothing, neither friends or enemies." Aristotle makes it clear that injuries and murders should take place between characters who are related by blood. Therefore, the most tragic plots would include fratricides, patricides, matricides etc., actions that would include recognitions immediately accompanied by reversals. These reversals are tied to the plots, for Aristotle stated that the best tragedies are those that proceed from inexplicably unreal plots, from which many actions could be derived.

- In the Oedipus example, the tragic fact is not that Oedipus killed a man, but that he killed his father. The recognition of the person, not the action or deed, is what was important in constructing Oedipus' reversal of fortune.

It is difficult for the reader to understand what Aristotle means when, in describing other forms of recognitions, he mentions "inanimate objects." Does he mean that although the recognition of things and events may be dramatic or exciting, this recognition cannot have tragic proportions of any magnitude, the way that a recognition of a person would have? When Oedipus recognized that Laius was his father, only after he had killed him, Oedipus progressed from ignorance to knowledge. Therefore, according to all the related arguments in the *Poetics,* the foundation of recognition is the knowledge of and the existence of the familial bond between two people. Aristotle is also preoccupied with the emotional effect that recognition, conjoined with reversal, would have on the audience. Both elements will engage the audience's emotions with "pity or with fear" because the audience will be aware of the reality of happiness or unhappiness.

Recognition will provoke pity only if that recognition occurs after the murder or fatal act, for Aristotle states in **Chapter Fourteen** that, " The better way for it to be done in ignorance, with the recognition following afterward," as in the case of Oedipus. Recognition will evoke fear, since it reveals the horror of the fatal act.

So, tragic recognition is the discovery of the identity of a blood related person after a fatal act, by a character who participates in this fatal act in a tragedy, who has already been defined in the plot as existing in a state of happiness or unhappiness. For Aristotle, as happiness and unhappiness are matters of knowledge, then the tragic hero's recognition involves self-knowledge, a primary reason for Aristotle rating recognition above reversal.

Aristotle later connects recognition to his structural analysis of the tragic plot and to the idea of tragic pathos (suffering) in *Chapters Thirteen and Fourteen*. Tragic recognition, while being a technical device, is, in its true essence, a powerful catalyst which provides an emotional rush, changing the audience's awareness of the realities within the tragedy. Both reversal and recognition represent unique methods in which tragic emotions, intrinsic to the structure of the tragedy's plot, are raised to heightened levels of intensity.

In *Chapter Ten,* Aristotle stated that pathos or suffering is not limited to complex plots. In Chapter Eleven, pathos is the fatal or painful event, that thing suffered, around which the action, simple or complex, revolves. Without pathos, the action would lack emotional intensity and potential.

This final element in **Chapter Eleven** includes a problem, centered on the idea that deaths should be "...in the open and not behind the scenes." The question arises as to whether he is talking about deaths and woundings occurring on stage. If he is directing that these events happen on stage, the <u>reader</u> of the tragedy would remain emotionally unaffected as he cannot react to this visual spectacle. Yet, Aristotle later states in Chapter Fourteen that "...anyone who merely hears the events unfold will shudder and feel pity as a result of what is happening." Here, Aristotle seems to resolve the troubling issue by stating that a mere narrative account of death or wounding, during the tragedy, will suffice to produce the desired emotional effects on its audience. The question still remains that since death, pain and wounding are visible events, can they have as much emotional effect by appearing as narrative events within the tragedy? Should they be made to appear as visible, physical events on stage, as part of a desired spectacle?

If only told through narrative, these fatal events would appear to weaken the argument that pathos, the third structural element of plot, is that event around which all action is centered. Pathos, then, would only be audibly visible, through the imagination of the audience, when it appears as a narrative component in the tragic plot, as a narrated point of reference to other events in the plot, an apparently abstract formulation on the part of Aristotle.

Works Cited

Else, Gerald F. *Aristotle's Poetics: The Argument.* Cambridge: Harvard University Press, 1963.

Grube, G.M.A. *Plato's Republic.* Indianapolis: Hackett Publishing Company, 1974.

Hutton, James. *Aristotle's Poetics,* an English Translation of the Poetics with Introduction and Notes. New York: Norton and Company, 1982.

Notes on *Aristotle's Poetics* the Arguments

Book 1: The Mimetic Arts

Introduction

- The art of poetry and its general nature.

- What characteristic effect poetry has.

- How plots should be constructed.

- The number and nature of the parts of each form.

The Basic principle: imitation

- Epic poetry, tragedy, comedy, the dithyramb and flute and lyre music are all imitations.

These differ by:

a.   using different means of imitation,

b.   imitating different objects,

c.   imitating in a different manner and mode.

Differences based on the means of imitation

- Just as painters make likenesses of objects by imitating their colors and forms, and actors imitate others by using their voice, then all the arts imitate through the <u>means</u> of rhythm, language and melody.

- These <u>means</u> can be used separately or together in various combinations.

- The art, which imitates language in prose, has no name.

- The word "poet" is attached to particular meters, such as elegiac and epic poets, not because of their type of imitation, but based on the meter they use.

- Anyone who produces an imitation, must, because of this imitation, be called a poet.

- Dithyrambic poetry (an elaborate choral song with narrative content), nomic poetry, tragedy and comedy use rhythm, song and metrical language.

    a. Dithyrambic and nomic employ all three media.

    b. Tragedy and comedy use different media.

Conclusion

- The forms of imitations are the means, the objects, and the manner of imitation.

- These forms produce the definitions of epic poetry, tragedy and comedy.

Aristotle's Poetics

I. Plot:

1. End result is *catharsis* (purging, relief of emotions)

2. *Plot* is an imtation of action

3. Parts of a plot:

    A. *Reversals* – change from one state of affairs to the opposite. Example: Poverty to riches or health to illness.

    B. *Recognitions* – change from ignorance to Knowledge; leads to friendship or hostility; Characters marked for good or bad fortune.

    C. *Suffering (pathos)* – destruction, pain, or death.

4. Qualities of a plot:

    A. *Completeness* – should not begin or end at a chance point in time

    B. *Magnitude – should be a length of time easily held in the memory. Must permit a change from bad* Fortune to good fortune or from good to bad Fortune.

5. Must represent the *universal in the particular.*

6. Types of plots:

   A. *Simple* – change of fortune without a reversal or Recognition.

   B. *Complex* – change of fortune involves a recognition or reversal or both.

7. Best plots:

   - Good people should not pass from From prosperity to misfortune.

   - Evil people should not rise from ill fortune to prosperity.

   - Characters should fail because of some mistake.

   - Story should affect pity and fear in the reader.

II. *Ordering of a plot:*

1. Study the *arrangement of incidents* in a plot; how the author arranges events:

   A. Chronological – in order of time

   B. Past – present – past

   C. Some plots begin at the end and lead up to why/how Events worked out.

   D. In medias res – in the middle of things

   E. Flashback – about events that happened before the opening scene.

2. *Exposition* – background info readers need to know to make sense of the situation in which the characters are placed.

3. *Rising action* – plot gains momentum; complications in the plot that intensifies situations.

4. *Conflict* – reveals characters/conveys meaning.

5. *Foreshadowing* – suggestion of what is to come.

6. *Protagonist* – hero, or central character; can be despicable as well as heroic.

7. *Antagonist* – force that opposes the protagonist.

8.   *Suspense* – makes reader uncertain and anxious about what is to come.

9.   *Climax* – moment of greatest emotional tension.

10.   *Resolution of conflict* – denouement (untying the knot).

Character:

1.   Characters are influenced by events, just as events are shaped by character. Characterization includes the idea that people in stories seem to actually exist; illusion of reality. Characters can be other than people.

2.   Author can reveal character by:

- *Names*: Can suggest a character's nature.
- *Physical description*: Clothing
- *Character*. Revealed by words/actions of those who respond to them.
- *Showing*: Reveal themselves by what they say or do.
- *Telling*: Economical descriptions.

3.   *Motivation* – reasons for behavior and speech.

4.   *Plausibility* – when adequate motivation is offered, the reader understands a character's actions, however bizarre.

5.   *Consistency* – behavior is compatible with details of temperment.

6.   In *absurdist literature* – characters are alienated from themselves and their environment in an irrational world. We find an antihero who has little control over events.

7.   *Dynamic characters* – undergo life changes because of the action of the plot.

8.   *Static characters* – do not change; often serve as a foil; reveal by contrast the distinctive qualities of another character.

9.   *Flat character* – embodies one or two qualities that can be summarized; one dimensional; not psychologically complex.

10.   *Stock* – stereotypes rather than indiviuduals.

11.   *Round* – more complex; have more depth of   personality; surprise or puzzle the reader.

Book 2: Differences Arising From the Objects Of Imitation

- Objects of imitation are people in action.

- People will either be of a higher (goodness) or lower (badness) moral type. Imitation of people by the poets is to be either better or worse than real people [in reality]. Sometimes the imitation will wholly be based upon reality and man will portrayed as he really is.

- Comedy imitates people who are worse than reality.

- Tragedy imitates people who are better than reality.

Book 3: Differences in the Manner of Imitating

- The manner of imitating objects (people) can be represented in the same medium but different modes.

- These modes include:

  a. Narration

  b. Dialogue (characters functioning and in action).

- The acting and doing mode (prattones and drontes):

  a. Doing (drontes)- Through this mode, the Dorians claimed to invent tragedy and comedy.

Book 4: The Origin Of Poetry And The Growth Of Drama

1. The origin of poetry has two causes:

   - Humans instinctively imitate. Man gets his first lessons through imitating others.

   - Humans take pleasure in imitating.

2. What is ugly or distressful in reality is seen with pleasure when depicted in realistic images.

3. The learning experience is pleasurable but limited. When realistic images are presented, people perceive through their reasoning abilities what each image represents. This gives them the pleasure of imitation. Unknown images, unable to be understood through ordinary perceptions, give pleasure on the basis of craftsmanship.

4.   Therefore, since imitation is a part of the human instinctive nature, people, adept at imitating rhythms and melodies, began creating poetry.

5.   Poetry split into:

- Serious souls began writing about noble actions and noble persons (tragedy),

- frivolous souls wrote about baser persons (comedy)

- Lampoons were written in iambic meter.

6.   Homer was a both a master of the serious, but was the first to use comedy by giving a dramatic approach to what was ridiculous.

7.   After the division of comedy and tragedy appeared, poets became either comic poets or tragic poets.

8.   Tragedy's origins were in improvisation through the dithyrambic chorus. Tragedy developed in dignity and its meter changes from the trochaic tetrameter (satyric, more oriented in dancing) to the iambic trimeter (most adept for speaking).

9.   Comedy's origins were in the phallic performances.

10. *Aeschylus* first increased the number of actors from one to two; reduced the importance of the chorus; made dialogue most important.

11. *Sophocles* added more actors and introduced scenery.

12. The poet-craftsman forms by experience more and more adequate notions (universals) of the form of tragedy, including a notion of magnitude as tragedy grew out of its initial small plots and ridiculous language into a sizable and solemn form attractive to serious poets.

Book 5: Notes on Comedy, Epic Poetry, and Tragedy

1.   Comedy is imitation of people who are worse than the average; steeped in the ridiculous or the shameful, which is not painful or destructive.

2.   History of comedy - origin of masks is unknown.

3.   Origin of comic plots came from Sicily.

4.   Crates in Athens was first to discard the abusive mode and construct universal plots.

5. Epic poetry came after tragedy and was an imitation of good men through metrical language.

6. Epic poetry and tragedy differ is that epic poetry uses narrative and a single meter, and is without restriction to time. Tragedy keeps "within one revolution of the sun." Tragedy uses music and spectacle and contains all the part of the epic. The epic, however, does not use all the parts that make up tragedy.

Appendix 5

This following is an unclassified response to questions posed at the Kent School

Dr. Deborah M. Coulter-Harris
27 October, 2000
Kent School of Analysis

The Cuba Snie
A Crucial Estimate Revisited

1. What were the shortcomings of the SNIE? What do you think of Kent's explanation of why the key judgment was wrong?

The SNIE failed to estimate Soviet deployment of missiles in Cuba. The SNIE centered on projecting political aspirations of Soviet policy makers and their Marxist allies in Cuba. While the SNIE did propose that there were Soviet weapons of a more offensive character being placed in Cuba, the SNIE's main military estimations concentrated on a military build-up indicating defensive capabilities rather than offensive intentions. The SNIE's worst case scenario was that Cuba would become more aggressive in its revolutionary activity in Latin America. More importantly, the SNIE miscalculated Soviet intent based upon established analytic perceptions of former Soviet practice and policy. Estimators were dubious that Soviets would increase a risk in US-Soviet relations.

Kent perceived that there had been either a neglect or misevaluation of evidence because it had not supported a preconceived hypothesis concerning Soviet intent; we did not believe that Khrushev could make a mistake; we had flawed insights into Soviet decision-making.

I support Kent's observations on other factors that contributed to analytic misjudgment. These observations include:

- The national estimates' board and staff were unable to read all incoming reports; information overload heightens human fallibilities relating to cognitive perceptions and ability to make sound judgment.

- People have inherent biases; some people actively resist new ideas.

- The mass of information received could have supported or destroyed almost any kind of hypothesis concerning the presence of strategic missiles.

- Aerial photography failed to spot the indicators of missile emplacement - made fools of ground observers by proving their reports inaccurate or wrong.

Information from U-2s etc., which could have verified Cuban missile sites and deployments, arrived after the estimate was completed. Kent proposes that if the estimate could have been recalled and modified, the most that could have been achieved was a softening of the original "highly unlikely" with a few added sentences to signal the possible emergence of a dangerous threat. Kent doubts that added information could have prompted the government to immediate action. Current intelligence becomes quickly dated; there is always a large GAP between long-range estimates, which rely on masses of current intelligence reports, and the volume of quick turn-around current intelligence, which relies on estimates for projections.

The estimators lacked direct evidence, and utilized only indicators mirror-imaging precedents in Soviet foreign policy. As Kent opines - it does not necessarily follow that you understand an enemy's probably behavior from this kind of approach; this only leads to a general understanding of a communist mindset but can never predict accurately the actions of a particular Soviet policy maker.

2. What could have been done to improve the Estimate?

Any attempt to re-estimate the original estimate concerning the Cuban missile fiasco would probably be an exercise in futility. I will only offer more philosophical suggestions to alter uncompromising and obdurate human cognitive processing operations. There must be recognition that a rigid acceptance of a singular purview on an intelligence situation will be flawed; analysts must always be prepared for an enemy's alternative behavior, and thus be prepared to reflect on alternative analyses.

The "treasure house" of previous analytic experiences regarding Soviet intentions was a type of subjectivity, which relegated the process of the comprehension of events in Cuba to a distortion of or disregard for certain aspects of likely Soviet intentions. An analyst may imagine the general intention of political and theoretical Marxists, but an analyst can never predict with certainty how particular Marxist politicians will respond to particular policies.

The ideal analyst should converge both historical and possible or likely perspectives on critical situations, thus forming an interaction of perspectives; this convergence of perspectives constructs a new type meaning guided by a more rational perspective of reality. Analysts should never react to their own "reality" solely based upon their own personal "storehouse" of experiences, which is called their "repertoire" (Iser 69).

This consists of everything that is familiar to an analyst who bases judgments on previous historical and contextual behaviors, respectively representational of thought systems, and past reactions to historical problems. New perspectives should be formed to construct an analysis that forms an interaction of perspectives that corrects deficiencies inherent in more rigid forms of analysis.

Appendix 6

Literary analysis of poetry with writing assignments.

Dr. Deborah M. Coulter-Harris

Cognitive Processing Operations

Readers are often frustrated by layered perspectives of a poetry text. The most complicated part of reading a piece of poetry, like any other type of reading, is the building of consistencies. Frustration often occurs between the narrator's repertoire and the personal repertoire the reader brings to the text. The reader's role is distinctly marked by her cognitive responses to the reading.

One way of building consistencies is to attempt to close the gaps in our reading of the author's text, text being anything from which we make meaning. The gaps a reader encounters are places in the text where the reader pauses to wonder how to make meaning, the place in the text where the reader lacks the information she needs to cognitively process the text. When gaps occur, we pause to wonder about the author's intent, and what the author means by various phrases and metaphors.

Our perspective of the author's text naturally affects our constructions of meaning. The sense we make of a text is dependent on our acculturated perspectives, and on our own special set of environmentally conditioned beliefs which are based upon our particular religious, political and economic circumstances.

Often, the theme we construct, as a response to a particular piece of reading, reflects our self-centered interests, so that we frequently find a theme, or make one, in reaction to the reading. We must also keep in mind the multiple possible responses, which are likely to occur when a multi-cultural audience of readers engages a text. The text then becomes the map on which the individual reader explores his potential responses.

The following poem, Emily Dickinson's "The Soul Selects Her Own Society," is presented here as an exploration into a woman's response to the world. The poem presents the reported action of how this woman's soul responds to the world. Now, being a Caucasian, Christian woman, who comes from the Massachusetts woods, as did Emily Dickinson, I want to build my own repertoire about what I could believe the speaker of the poem means. What are the things I know about the text of the poem, which lie outside its content, on which I could build my own personal text? How am I going to achieve consistency in my response by closing the gaps I see between my repertoire and the text the author has presented?

The cognitive complexities derived from my reading of the poem will rely on the level of my critical competency, on my critical literacy as a reader. Within the academic discipline of aesthetic response, the cognitive processes I engage in will come from the source, Dickinson's poem, and will be fashioned in response to the following four cognitive processing categories (Stein 121-123).

1.) As the readers observe what Dickinson has written, they should attempt to comprehend the poetess' words. This will be the first task, that of **monitoring,** that is, how will you build your response to the text?

2.) The readers should then try to **elaborate** on the text, producing new meaning, in order to enhance both the text of the poem, and their own personal text which they have set out to produce as a response to the author's utterances. This stage involves the reader's own repertoire of knowledge, and their competence in using their cognitive processing abilities. Here, the reader's prior knowledge combines with the source text to create new propositions, ideas and critical perspectives. This is the move from reading to writing, the beginning of the creation of the reader's written response text.

3.) The reader as writer now proceeds onto the **structuring** phase of her cognitive response to the text. Here, the readers must determine how to shape or reshape the material they have gathered. At this stage, the readers/writers manipulate new propositions in the source text to create a text of their own. The readers here decide what propositions they agree or disagree with, and arrange these propositions into categories, according to their cognitive complexities. Here the writer should attempt to discover relations between the various propositions of the text, and her own textual response to them, constructing categories which are hierarchal, in descending subordinate positions, that is, from the cognitively complex to the cognitively less complex.

4.) The **planning** or shaping stage of the writing process now commences, as the reader/writer deals with the contextual ideas in the source text, or from those ideas in the text which connect to the writer's memory. Here we must develop those organizing ideas, that will logically guide the construction of the reader's personal response text. It is at this phase of the readers' cognitive processing that they develop their sense of a rhetorical purpose in order to make meaning.

Let's begin reading "The Soul Selects Her Own Society" below:

The soul selects her own society,
Then shuts the door;
On her divine majority
Obtrude no more.

Unmoved, she notes the chariot's pausing
At her low gate;
Unmoved, an emperor is kneeling
Upon her mat.

I've known her from an ample nation
Choose one;
Then close the valves of her attention
Like stone.

Writing Assignment

Please respond to the above poem through the four cognitive processing techniques that have just been elaborated on. Attempt to write about the poem using the following questions as guides to assemble your responses:

1. What is Dickinson saying about the soul? Why has the author chosen to make the soul gendered? Is the author talking about her personal soul or about the universal soul of mankind?

2. What connotations constitute the word "divine?" What defines the author's perspective of the "divine?" How does her soul, and the society she has selected, connect to this idea of divinity? Is the author writing in a biblical or prophetic tradition? If so, why did she pick this particular genre of writing to get her idea of divinity across to the reader?

3. As a reader, you will probably experience a gap in your understanding of the term "chariot." Is the author connecting the utterance to the world of gods and goddesses who move through the sky in the Greek tradition? Or does this word refer to the Chariots of Israel which the prophet Elijah rode on during his journey from earth to heaven? How would either reference change the poem's meaning? How would your selection build consistency of meaning according to the author's intent? What do think a "low-gate" is? Why is the chariot "pausing" there?

4. Whom do you think the "emperor" is representative of? Why is he kneeling on her mat? What kind of mat can this be? Is the Emperor at her door? What can you make of the fact that both the chariot and the emperor are respectively pausing and kneeling close to her?

5. The speaker describes the woman coming from an "ample nation." Why do you think this woman has been imbued with the qualities of strength and honor?

6.   When the woman selects, she selects selectively the society in which she wants to live. She boldly closes off all other societies. Her wishes appear to engraved in stone, as she "closes the valves of her attention, like stone?"

     A. What does the utterance "stone" mean to you? Does this word continue the consistency of the prophetic tradition?

     B. How can your religious or your literary repertoire help you to understand the multiple representations of the author's meanings?

     C. How big are "the valves of attention" of which the narrator speaks? Can everyone close these valves, or is it only the soul which remains unmoved, by a chariot or by the appearance of an emperor, which is able to close these valves?

     D. Why do you think the author selected the word "valves?"

     Let's move to a second poem by Emily Dickinson entitled, "My Life Closed Twice Before Its Close." Once again, respond to the poem by using the four cognitive processing techniques based upon the questions following the poem.

My life closed twice before its close;
It yet remains to see
If immortality unveil
A third event to me,

So huge, so hopeless to conceive,
As these that twice befell.
Parting is all we know of heaven,
And all we need of hell.

Writing Assignments

1.   What are the gaps presented which delay your full understanding of the poem? What is your perception of death? What do you anticipate about death?

2.   What is the speaker's conception of death, and how does she understand and anticipate it? Why is her perception of death "huge, helpless to conceive?" In your understanding of what is sublime versus what is beautiful, what aspects of death are sublime or beautiful according to the speaker of the poem? Does the speaker believe that death is religiously or spiritually terrifying? Are you able to conceive of another kind of life dimension beyond this material life?

3.	Dickinson makes the point that we know nothing more about heaven than that we must part from the earth to get there. Now the speaker of the above poem has stated that her life closed two times before her life ended. However, she is still alive when she makes this statement. Can there be other kinds of death in life than our own physical death? Can you construct what kinds of deaths these are? If the speaker is talking about her personal tragedies, how does this change the meaning of the poem?

4.	Is all you need to know of hell the experience of a loved one dying? Have you ever lost anyone close to you? How did you feel? How did you personally respond to their death? How does your response to death connect to the author's response? To what degree are you happy on this earth, or to what degree are you afraid of the "immortality of death?"

5.	In response to the author's idea of heaven and hell, what are your conceptions of these sublime places? Are your ideas of heaven and hell contingent upon some kind of personal religious training? If so, how does your religious background hinder or help in terms of your understanding what the poem means?

6.	Can we experience a type of heaven and hell on earth? Please describe a personal life experience that was happy, or one that was very sad. Can you relate this experience to the possible experiences the author might have had which prompted her responding to death, and heaven and hell in the way she did?

Writing to Connect Self with Others

Now that you have explored Emily Dickinson's ideas on the divinity of the soul and on different types of death, and now that you have built some consistencies in your mind regarding the author's intent, as well as your own personal response and understanding of the concepts presented in the texts of the two poems, you will select one of the following essay topics:

1.	Both poems deal with a form of spiritual response to the world we must live in. The speaker of the first poem has her "soul" selecting the society in which it chooses to live. It may appear that Dickinson believes we determine our own lives, in opposition to some, who believe that our lives are determined by circumstances beyond our control. Narrate a personal story that deals with a particular circumstance in your life that was beyond your control. How did this situation affect or control other areas of your life? Alternatively, narrate a story about a time in your life when you were able to successfully control a personal life situation which, at first, seemed out of your control.

2. Think about a time when you lost someone close to you. Narrate a story about this person, explaining how this person influenced your life. In this story, describe your feelings and reaction to this person's death. How did the death affect your life and your thinking about life?

3. You may also choose to write about an event in your life that was as difficult to handle emotionally as the death of a loved one. Describe how this event changed the circumstances and direction of your life. How was this event like a death to you?

Appendix 7

The Infamous Declassified PDB

Declassified and Approved
for Release, 10 April 2004

Bin Ladin Determined To Strike in US

Clandestine, foreign government, and media reports indicate Bin Ladin since 1997 has wanted to conduct terrorist attacks in the US. Bin Ladin implied in US television interviews in 1997 and 1998 that his followers would follow the example of World Trade Center bomber Ramzi Yousef and "bring the fighting to America."

After US missile strikes on his base in Afghanistan in 1998, Bin Ladin told followers he wanted to retaliate in Washington, according to a ███████████████ service.

An Egyptian Islamic Jihad (EIJ) operative told an ███████ service at the same time that Bin Ladin was planning to exploit the operative's access to the US to mount a terrorist strike.

The millennium plotting in Canada in 1999 may have been part of Bin Ladin's first serious attempt to implement a terrorist strike in the US. Convicted plotter Ahmed Ressam has told the FBI that he conceived the idea to attack Los Angeles International Airport himself, but that Bin Ladin lieutenant Abu Zubaydah encouraged him and helped facilitate the operation. Ressam also said that in 1998 Abu Zubaydah was planning his own US attack.

Ressam says Bin Ladin was aware of the Los Angeles operation.

Although Bin Ladin has not succeeded, his attacks against the US Embassies in Kenya and Tanzania in 1998 demonstrate that he prepares operations years in advance and is not deterred by setbacks. Bin Ladin associates surveilled our Embassies in Nairobi and Dar es Salaam as early as 1993, and some members of the Nairobi cell planning the bombings were arrested and deported in 1997.

Al-Qa'ida members—including some who are US citizens—have resided in or traveled to the US for years, and the group apparently maintains a support structure that could aid attacks. Two al-Qa'ida members found guilty in the conspiracy to bomb our Embassies in East Africa were US citizens, and a senior EIJ member lived in California in the mid-1990s.

A clandestine source said in 1998 that a Bin Ladin cell in New York was recruiting Muslim-American youth for attacks.

We have not been able to corroborate some of the more sensational threat reporting, such as that from a ███████████████ *service in 1998 saying that Bin Ladin wanted to hijack a US aircraft to gain the release of "Blind Shaykh" 'Umar 'Abd al-Rahman and other US-held extremists.*

continued

For the President Only
6 August 2001

Declassified and App
for Release, 10 Apri

The above PDB was originally published before 9/11 and warned of a Bib Ladin attack; The CIA had once again done its job of warning.

Appendix 8

Source Evaluation Form

Source Evaluations
Dr. Coulter-Harris

(You must fill out and complete one evaluation for every source you use.)

1. Title of Source:

2. Author:

3. Date of publication:

4. Derivation of source (Internet, library, academic journal, magazine etc.):

5. Host of Internet site:

6. Date you downloaded source:

7. **Edition or Revision**:

8. **Publisher**:

9. **Title of Journal**:

10. Is the Information Accurate?

    • Are facts and statistics verifiable?

    • Is there a bibliography?

11. **Is the Information Objective?**

    • Is there any noticeable bias?

12. **Is the Information Current?**

    • Is this the most current information on your topic?

13. Full MLA Citation of

Source:_____

_____

_____

_____

14. Summary of Source (attach typed summary to form):

15. What Main Points in your paper will this source

Appendix 9

Global Topics

Dr. Coulter-Harris

I. Topics for Paper #1: Political Commentary

You may select from any of the following topics for your first paper:

1. Examine the **role of women in any of the great religions** – Hinduism, Islam, Judaism, and Christianity. Which religion allows women the greatest access to power? Which religion allows women the least access? What are the social and political ramifications of denying women equal rights and political power in repressive societies?

2. Is imperialistic activity justified when a country suffers from a lack of a **certain resource?** Use examples of imperialistic activity from past and recent political events. Has the recent war in Iraq strengthened or weakened the U.S. economy? Why are Iraqis paying a nickel a gallon for gasoline while gas skyrockets in the U.S.?

3. **Global Warming. – hype or reality?** There is a great debate—mainly political—that global warming is changing weather patterns, affecting crops and economies etc. There are other scientists who say that global warming does not exist because earth's weather patterns have always been in a continual state of change. Take a position.

4. **Agro-terrorism.** How do we stop terrorists from poisoning our crops and food supplies? Do you see this situation as a real or imagined threat?

5. The move toward **globalization** has brought ensuing economic disasters in third world countries, and intensified the unification of national and religious identities. **Is it futile to assume that the United States can impose globalized democratic ideals upon Islamic civilizations that reject American cultural imperialism?**

6. Recent national and international trends support the hypothesis that **our historical tradition of the democratic-secular state is being replaced with the politics of religious rhetoric and faith-based political initiatives**, which will diminish our capacity to influence democratic ideals in foreign policy initiatives. The rise and influence of Christian fundamentalist ideology on national leaders in our own country undermines the very basis of our concept of separation of church and state.

- While we seek moral, just, and wise leadership in the United States, will the rise of theocratic politicians pandering to select religious communities exacerbate religious differences in our own country and provoke foreign governments on whom we must negotiate for resources?

7. **Examine the role of women in any of the great religions** – Hinduism, Islam, Judaism, and Christianity. Which religion allows women the greatest access to power? Which religion allows women the least access? What are the political and social ramifications of denying women equal social and political power within a society?

8. **Human beings have a collective unconsciousness about their true origins.** Research Zecharia Sitchin's theories about the origins of the human race in <u>The Earth Chronicles.</u> How would his theories topple existing religious establishments? Would his theories unite or further divide the world?

9. **U.S. Trade deficit with China and India.** Will these countries replace America as economic world leaders?

10. **Patriot Act** – Protecting citizens from terrorism or abusing U.S. citizens constitutional rights?

11. **AIDs in Africa** – Does the West really care that AIDs is decimating the African continent?

12. **Nuclear weapons development in North Korea** – Why should we care if North Korea has nuclear weapons? Is there a solution to the problem?

13. Palestinians should/should not have a homeland.

14. **Iraq situation – heading towards democracy or civil war?** Will Iraq become a fundamentalist Shia (theocratic) state? Will there be civil war? If so, explain the paradox of U.S. efforts in Iraq.

15. **Iran situation** – should US invade and overthrow Ayatollahs to prevent Iran from gaining nuclear weapons that threaten Israel?

16. **Terrorists are seeping through the Mexican and Canadian borders.** What should be done to prevent this problem?

17. **Our major television news stations are propaganda arms of the United States government.** U.S. citizens receive only selective news items that divert attention away from real issues.

Appendix 10

Divergent/Convergent Thinking

Step 1: Divergent: Brainstorm
Step 2: Convergent: Winnow and cluster
Step 3: Convergent: Select practical, promising ideas

Divergence

- Branch out in different directions

- Opens mind to new ideas and creative alternatives

Convergence

- Bringing together and moving toward a point

- Views a problem more narrowly until it produces a single solution

- Winnows out the weak alternatives and chooses the strong

- Helps bring problem solving to closure

Brainstorm

- Means more than just discuss; should be freewheeling process of generating ideas randomly and spontaneously without worry about their practicality

Four Commandments of Divergent Thinking

- The more ideas, the better

- Build one idea upon the other

- Wacky ideas are okay; help break out of conventional thinking

- Don't evaluate ideas – this liberates people from self-imposed restraints in generating ideas

Apply 3-step divergent/convergent technique:

- Write as many remedies to the problem as you can think of

- Winnow and cluster ideas into categories

- Select ideas that are intuitively practical and promising

Appendix 11

Analytic Methods Example: Pre-Writing Exercise Example

Dr. Deborah M. Coulter-Harris

How Will the Russian Government Deal With Consortium Members?

It would be impossible to predict accurately how the Russian government would deal with the International Space Station's Consortium members. The evidence provided is restricted to the financial and technological failure of the Russian Space Program and to Russia's inability to provide technological services on time to the International Space Station. No evidence is provided relating to the historical partnership amongst Consortium members, and no facts are offered indicating or proving that Russia would definitively react in a surreptitious or predictive manner.

It would be possible to engage in prophetic analysis, which would offer, at best, semi- specious and speculative propositions, derived from neither deductive nor inductive formulation:

- The Russians might miraculously come up with the redesign of the docking mechanism and meet their six-month tardy deadline.

- The Russians might ask for an extension of their deadline, citing technological difficulties.

- The Russians could resign from the Consortium and save face, citing a number of reasons:

  - Incompatibility with the US or with France or with England;

  - Realignment of a new Consortium with China or other countries. Etc.

- The Russians could come clean, explain their technological problems, and ask for scientific aid and further funding.

- The Russians might ask for technological assistance, forming a new alliance with private American or European industries.

- The Russians could resign from the Consortium without offering any explanation.

Etc.

How I Arrived at My Findings

It could be argued that this assignment begged for an alternative analysis; however, inherent in the construction of an alternative analysis is the existence of a conventional analysis with all of its constituent parts – hypothesis, evidence, and derived deductive or inductive conclusions. *There is no evidence provided in the written material concluding that the Russian government would react to the Consortium in any particular way.*

An examination of the data from the first paragraph provided urges the reader to construct a classical deductive syllogism. The specific conclusion derived offers no evidence of how Russia will deal with Consortium members.

Major Premise: A successful space program must have adequate funds and human scientific expertise.

Minor Premise: Russia's space program lacks adequate funding and human expertise.

Conclusion: The Russian space program is a failure.

An examination of the second paragraph provided calls for the analyst to reason inductively, drawing a general conclusion from an array of specific facts. The conclusion again offers no insight into Russia's intentions towards Consortium members.

Conclusion: The delivery of supplies and crews to the International space station will not arrive on time.

Evidence: The docking mechanism for the Russian shuttlecraft is flawed and requires:

- redesign.

- The redesign will delay deliveries by 12 months.

- The delivery is already six months behind schedule.

An examination of the final paragraph offers the following speculative conclusion based upon one lone piece of evidence leading to tenuous inductive reasoning. This particular conclusion, however, offers no evidence of how Russia will deal with consortium members and is based upon probability and not certainty.

Conclusion: Russia could be dropped from the Space Consortium if its latest technical problem is revealed.

Evidence: Consortium members have recommended that Russia's Consortium membership be dropped because of past delays and problems.

The major conclusion that we have been asked to provide, namely, that Russia will deal with the Consortium members in such and such a way, is *impossible to determine from the evidence provided.* The three derived conclusions

- the Russian space program is a failure

- the delivery of supplies and crews will not arrive on time

- *Russia could be dropped from the program*

are not relational to the problem posed, and do not in any way offer cogent insight into Russia's intentions or future actions towards the Consortium.

Appendix 12

Example of Decision Tree Logic (Jones 125-126)

The Decision Event Tree

A decision event tree is a diagram that graphically shows <u>choices and their outcomes</u> at different junctures in alternative sequences or chains of events.

Figure 1: The Lady or the Tiger

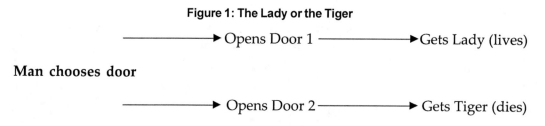

The tree portrays two alternative scenarios, or sequences of events.

Scenario A: Chooses door – opens Door 1 – gets lady (lives).
Scenario B: Chooses door – opens Door 2 – gets tiger (dies).

This example demonstrates the two immutable, universal characteristics of a decision/tree event:

- The branches of the tree are *mutually exclusive*, meaning that, if the actor (person making the choice) picks door 1, he can't also pick door 2.

- The branches are *collectively exhaustive*, meaning that the alternatives at each branch incorporate all possibilities; no other options (other decisions or events) are possible at that point in the sequence or scenario.

Figure 2: Make a Purchase

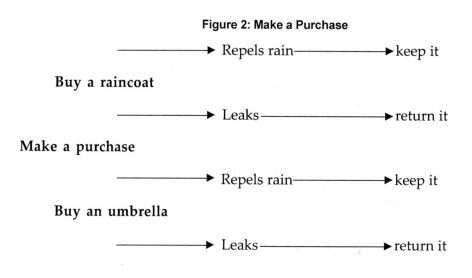

The decision tree scenario enables us to structure analysis of a problem:

- Dissects scenario into sequential events.

- Shows cause-and-effect linkages.

- Shows which decisions or events are dependent on others.

- Shows where linkages are strongest and weakest.

- Enables us to visually compare how one scenario differs from another.

- Reveals alternatives we might not perceive and enables us to analyze them

Four steps in Constructing a Decision Event Tree:

- Identify the problem

- Identify the major factors/issues (the decisions and events) to be addressed in the analysis.

- **Identify alternatives for each of these factors/issues.**

- **Construct a tree portraying all alternative scenarios.**

These instructions are based upon Morgan D. Jones' instructions in *The Thinker's Toolkit*. New York: Random House, 1998, 125-126.

Appendix 13

Handwritten: Appendix 1 for arg paper

Hypothesis Testing and Matrix Chart[1]

Handwritten: AH. Hypothesis Testing Matrix

Hypothesis Testing

Dr. Deborah Coulter-Harris

We assert the truth of a hypothesis by offering supporting evidence. We disapprove a hypothesis with evidence. When we find "evidence," we should try to establish its validity by answering four questions:

- Who or what was the source?

- What was the source's access?

- What is the source's reliability?

- Is the information plausible? Make sense? Common or rare?

Figure 1. Hypothesis Testing Matrix

Evidence	Hypothesis A	Hypothesis B	Hypothesis C
1.			
2.			
3.			
4.			

Eight Steps of Hypothesis Testing:

1. Generate hypothesis.

2. Construct a matrix. Label the first column "Evidence."

3. List "significant" evidence down the left-hand margin, including absent evidence.

4. Working across the matrix, test the evidence for consistency with each hypothesis, one item of evidence at a time. Determine whether the evidence is consistent (C), inconsistent (I), or ambiguous (?). Consistency

---

1 These instructions are based upon Morgan D. Jones' instructions in *The Thinker's Toolkit*. New York: Random House, 1998, Chapter 11.

does not mean the evidence necessarily validates the hypothesis. It means the evidence is compatible with the hypothesis. In the case of inconsistency, the hypothesis could not be true, given the evidence. You may indicate varying degrees of consistency with – or +.

5. Refine the matrix. Add or reword hypothesis. Add "significant" evidence relevant to any new or reworded hypothesis and test it against all hypotheses.

6. Working downward, evaluate each hypothesis. Delete any hypothesis for which there is significant inconsistent evidence. Re-evaluate and confirm the validity of inconsistent evidence.

7. Rank the remaining hypothesis by the weakness of inconsistent evidence. The hypothesis with the weakest inconsistent evidence is the most likely.

8. Perform a sanity check.

Hypothesis Testing Matrix

Evidence	Hypothesis A	Hypothesis B	Hypothesis C

Appendix 14

Individual Reasearch Project (IRP) Evaluation Chart

Name: xxxxxxxxxxxx

IRP: *Global Warming*

Section	Excellent	Very Good	Good	Fair	Poor	Incomplete
Research Proposal	+					
Graphic Cover Page	+					
CONTENTS	+					
Abstract	+					
Letter of Transmittal	+					
Key Findings	+					
Major Headers	+					
Minor Headers	+					
Use of Bullets	+					
Analysis	+					
Analytic Transitions	+					
Use of Graphics	+					
Captions	+					
OUTLOOK: F.I.	+					
Overall Presentation	+					
APPENDIX 1.	+					
Appendix 2. Extended Definition	+					
Glossary	+					
NOTES	+					
Sources: Parenthetical Citations	+					
Works Cited	+					
Brochure	+					
Source Evaluations	+					
Final Analysis of Project	+					
Self-Analysis	+					
PowerPoint Presentation	+					

Paper: Your IRP was exceptional. Your writing, presentation, and execution are excellent. I am pleased with your overall presentation. Your major and minor headers were analytic and in active voice, and your analytic statements drew the reader to the paper. The Portfolio was well-organized; your paper was very well-written with few or no edits or corrections. The structure of the paper was perfect. Graphics were outstanding, and captions were well-written and professional. Overall, the project was very well executed with very strong analysis.

- **Your Key Findings were succinct and would give a busy executive the information needed to assess the report.** Your use of evidentiary bullets was excellent and reflected the expanse of the research and conclusions in the paper. Your OUTLOOK was strong and professional.

- The time and effort you spent on this project was exemplary. The writing improvements you show in this paper are indicative of your attention to details and to my instructions.

Appendix 15

Poems: I am including some past poems already published

"The First Light"

I was 7, an age of reason,
With Nazarite hair and pure complexion,
Walking from Mary Jane's house, the sun
low upon our hills. Suddenly, a comet
at four o'clock, flew over my head. I bet
I could touch that light -
It had landed! Many nights
had I lived in the unseen, and unafraid,
yet curious, I called Rose to tell her:
" I have seen the sun fall in the afternoon.
It tumbled onto your hill, or got buried in the timber."

All the children fell to search.
No deeply graven hole held this angel light.
Nor did we unearth in our thick birch,
richly-wrapped homes, that we were divine -
that would come later.

" Four Movements of a Connemara Queen"

1.

After long journeys
the old woman sits to rest
her elbow on her walking stick,
brown, beaten, whittled by the wind.
Her home is where the homeless have slept,
flats in a literary town,
flats in an illiterate town,
homes by the sea,
hostels made of salt and wind.

The log, her chair,
where some cutter axed his firewood
rises splintered to her flesh
but she perceives no jabs.
Seasons are more distinct
Time, stars and sun.
She arises from trenches, caves, cottages, castles
to snap new moons into sight
that she may live the month.

" The way the key fitted the door
heavy it was with string around my neck,
orange, pale apricot knotting
was like the way he fitted me.
Time left me locked
a broken hinge left for the wind to rattle."

2.

After long rests
the old woman stands
her hand melting about the stick handle
pat and step, pat step, pat step
the valley has no echo to her movement.
Passing old stone fences
hanging on the mountainside
like cobwebs on a wall,
old rocks which fortified old towns, now gone,
they sailed away before they died.

" Memories of Jack the Idiot,
slow learner the villagers decided,
was strong as seven men.
Saw two swans sailing across the bay
said he would be leaving them.
The villagers joked.
The joke of the village died that night
in a fever that set the bay to boiling."

3.

" What's the time?" he asked. " Midnight."
That way she worried about the trees that summer,
late months of summer when the ferns curl brown
as if they were burnt. They were.
When the leaves, blown,
crackle at the door's empty space
everything burnt.

Rowen berries had fallen like apples,
the house trimmed with these magic berries of good fortune,
All the trees,
that way she feared them without their dress.
" The holly bush would remain," she thought.

What posture should she, can she take
what way to dream asleep?
" I sleep with arms around trees,
smooth ones, the way his skin was golden then
as if I were stroking the side of the sun."

4.

Not tired,
the old woman feels the ghosts roaming the bog.
By night, scents of heather, mists that smell of princes, peasants.
By day, blocks of earth dug, piled brown
wet fortresses of sheep, flowers, men
now warmth for the open hearth.

When firesmoke filled the room
like fog on the bay,
friends sitting, smoking, piping, barely visible
poteen eyed, bleary bright talk.
Then would she sings the three songs
that she knew by heart,
three love songs:
a warning, a waiting, and a wooing.

" The Lord's Island "

Lord Rupert Revelstoke lived on Lambay Island
in a castle, fortified by walls. From the beach
in Rush, I called to the gods that some fisherman's hand
would weaken, needing help. I needed to reach
Lambay's shore. Without praying much more,
I ran Main Street down, past twelve pubs to the docks,
and saw Thomas McGhee, a salty old sea hawk.
His rift was solid with lobsters and crabs.
I begged him to sail me to Lambay's rocks.

Our day-trip began slitting mackerel and tying
dead bodies to the lobster traps' eyes
which would seek out red-speckled, lazy sea-monsters.
When remote from the sheltered shore, having tossed
pots into the incorrigible currents, a heaving moss
of bulbous seaweed was captured. At a loss
to know what creatures we had fathomed, I struggled
and towed the sea's treasure to the boat's wet bottom.
I screamed at the horror the cage had unveiled.
A gigantic sea snake, a scummy, Caucasian conger eel.

I threw up my hands,
the pot crashed to the deck.
McGhee drew out his knife
and cut off the neck
of this rabid sea dog,
and threw the choice carcass into a pot,
the final graveyard for the ocean's caught.
When, after ample draughts of spirits and poteen,
our boiled feast of sea snake, meat white and lean,
lusciousness of lobster, flesh of the under seas,
I marveled that the Irish Sea had furnished me
so freely, feeding and sustaining this wandering company.

One night at midnight, Thomas and I had made a pact
to tour Lambay Island. We had to be secret, the fact
of our meeting and sailing under a full moon
would seem to Rush's townsfolk to be soon
an engagement or a wedding. They could gossip

and talk as they liked. I was a mere twenty-two
and Thomas McGhee, a wizened though handsome man,
almost toothless, could never have won my hand.

Our old lobster boat ploughed the kelp and jelly fish,
the smell of brine and salt, and those seal guards, a hoard,
an army protecting the Lord's mysterious shore.
Our vessel veered against the strip of tan sand
and scraped upon the salted strand, a muffled scream
heralding these buccaneers' landings, a mystical dream.

Directly I would discern the differences between kings
and commoners, between lords and peasants, that those wings
of chance and birth would sear my social self-esteem,
and in self-knowledge of lowly birth, despite those beams
and flashes of paradisal light, I knew that I was poor.
That one man could own so much, vast portions of fish
and flesh and birds and land, I could not understand.

Thomas and I, hand in hand,
whispered silently to the band
of miniature horses
at the first gate to the first field.
They were a freak of nature
or of man's breeding skills.
Still, with bloodshot eyes
and platinum manes, they thrilled
at their wet, bedraggled invaders.
A wall soon met us, as high
as the gulls fly,
but its sides were built in steps
so that any uninvited guest
could climb and scale the depths
within the Lord's sumptuous paradise.

I thought that my heart would burst,
bloody within, but soon Thomas and I
had made our way into a doorway,
then a hall. I called
to Thomas. I was deathly afraid.
Thomas had the gall

to steal food from the Lord's kitchen.
Breads and meats,
cheeses and fruits,
eggs and milk,
fine wines and sweets,
a god-like treat
we quickly conveyed outdoors.

On an archery gallery,
we celebrated and chuckled, barely
aware of the bursting blue moon,
of the tearing tides
stranding us on the Lord's fortress until dawn.

We hid
beneath nocturnal silence,
the muzzled sounds of snoozing
beasts, a drowsy feral ritual of nature.
A fiery flame bid
these buccaneers bolt
from a dreamlit voyage, their venture
ending with a light,
exposing these intrepid trespassers
as nomadic knights
in quest of a revelation so vast, past
wisdom threw up its hands and said, "There are many who
have searched for truth, but none so avariciously as you."

Reason then roared off the walls and into the streets
that riches and poverty are governed by chance, not feats
of talent nor hard work nor sweat, but through stable seats
of ancestry, an antithesis to my absurd American dream.

We fell forward
into the crusty old lobster boat,
the rising tide
heaving the aging ark into a tempest.
We were not tossed, we were in flight,
the swells coating
our skin, our vestments unearthly white.
I sat nestled

on the middle timber
while Thomas stood at the stern,
our guide through our concluding confrontation. He turned
the creaking craft through curling whitecaps of death,
and a drowning half the Irish Sea's gaping mouth imagined.

I remember howling and stamping my feet.
I was invincible.
I would will this hurricane to halt,
hold its breath,
while Thomas and his pirate queen
were delivered from death.

There were many who missed us,
the talk of the town.
We were met by the locals with food,
beer and frowns.
We were scolded,
rebuked and reproved for our venture,
a routine bourgeois response
reserved for explorers
who return with no plunder,
no spoils, no booty, no gifts.

As a stranger,
desiring that neither quarrels nor rifts
would rupture Rush's social harmony, I quietly stated,
" Thomas and I have seen the isolation
of the Lord, his fate reserved in abject desolation,
a lonely island for a lonely man."

" Starbuck Sings for the Lady"

" I will have no man in my boat,"
said Starbuck,
" who is not afraid of a whale."
An old man offers conversation.
His hands cannot bend circular
to tell what suffering has been.
He knew the distances it takes to run away,
what star to hide behind, how much to pay.

" The leaves have turned to scarlet
the leaves are burning gold.
Black fears I left in Dublin
Black fears I still behold.
White flesh, in turn, is aged
White flesh is new again.
Three apples for your graces
      and I'm growing."

His fantasies are exiled to the Sunday Supplement,
no gods are raised in his image.
He has seen Achilles without regrets
he's seen Achilles smoking cigarettes.
Prophesies are not wasted on his notions,
Analysis replaces mythology,
and he's left to his own transformations.

" The leaves have turned to scarlet
the leaves are burning gold.
Black fears I left in Dublin
Black fears I still behold.
White flesh, in turn, is aged
white flesh is new again.
Three apples for your graces
      and I'm growing."

Appendix 16

"The Hanging Gardens of Babylon"
by: Dr. Deborah Coulter-Harris

Forward to the Word Opera and about the author

Ancient History Background

I have been interested in World Religion and ancient religious scriptures all of my life; it has been my passion, despite long venues in other academic disciplines and employments. I studied acting at the *Abbey* and *Gates* theaters when I was a young actress in *Dublin, Ireland*; worked later as speechwriter to Mr. L.J. Sevin, former CEO of *Mostek Corporation* in *Dallas*; served in the *United States Army*; taught English, Math and U.S. History courses to United States Army soldiers in *Drama, Greece,* and, at the same time, taught English to Greek students at *Anglika Mavromatis*; taught at colleges and universities in Ohio, New York, and Philadelphia, and served as a *Middle East political analyst at C.I.A.* In January, 2005, I published my second collection of poetry, *Freed from the Plough and Other Innocent Tales,* with Tyborne Hill Publishers in California; my first small poetry collection, *The Dirt Road,* was published in 1976, by *Manloc Press in Dublin, Ireland.* I wrote the manuscript of this opera, *The Hanging Gardens of Babylon,* during June and July 2005.

I have found one single unifying element in all the major religions on earth today—every patriarch and prophet from all earth's major existing religions—all were visited by beings from the sky, who were linguistically anointed as *angels* and *gods*. The very first mention of these beings is in the Sumerian *Atra-Hasis Epic,* an ancient Babylonian account of the Great Deluge, when the Eden of the *Bible* became "a brackish desolate plain. As the epic states, there was mass starvation, disease became rampant, and the survivors had to resort to cannibalism." This condition was imposed by the "gods" of ancient Sumer, who found human numbers and noise disturbing. In the Sumerian *The Epic of Gilgamesh,* the deluge was decided by the ancient serpent [or dragon] gods in counsel. [1]

The original Anunn'aki father god was called *Anu* or "Sky"[2], the highest of the Mesopotamian gods; *Enki* was the male head of earth, and *Ninshursaga*[3] was a goddess and producer of life, equal but partially subordinate to Anu, Enki, and Enlil, Enki's brother. According to E.O.James, "Under the leadership of Anu, the god of heaven, whose name means 'sky,' 'shining,' 'bright,' the cosmic order was

---

1   R.A. Boulay's *Flying Serpents and Dragons.* Escondido: The Book Tree, 1999, 97, 99.

2   E.O. James. *The Ancient Gods.* New Jersey: Castle Books, 1999, 69, 73.

3   This spelling is one of several

established... from the time of *Gudea*, the priest of *Lagash* (c. 2060-2042 BC) he became supreme. ...even after his cult had fallen into obscurity....his supremacy was affirmed and maintained, and in the later theological lists of gods he always stood at the head." Anu's son Enlil was the Storm-god and King of gods, [4] and, as James writes, "He became the great Sumerian deity, the leader of the pantheon during the greater part of the third millennium B.C[5]....Enlil was the executor of divine power on earth from time immemorial."[6] The third member of the male Triad was Enki, sometimes called EA, who lived beneath the earth underground or in dark places like forests; he was reportedly kindly, wise, and taught humans writing and geometry.

Most Religions Employ Dragon Images

Most of the world's religious and ancient historical traditions are rooted in the serpent or the dragon tradition. The Chinese claim ancestry from their *Dragon gods*, and have the *Dragon* as their national symbol, as does Singapore. According to R.A. Boulay, "In earlier days, Asian dragons shared the world with humankind and did so peacefully...According to Chinese history, the first humans were believed to have been created by an ancient goddess named *Nu Kua*, who was herself part dragon and part mortal."[7] This is fairly similar in detail to the creation of the first Adam by the Anunn'aki dragon goddess, *Ninharsag*, the Chief Medical Officer of the original Anunn'aki, who performed genetic manipulation of Anunn'aki genes and those of a native earth hominid to produce the first "man," as detailed in the *King List, Book of Enoch,* and ancient Sumerian texts. According to the ancient *Book of Dzyan*, the oldest of Indian *Sanskit* sources, the Sumerians, led by Enki, colonized Mohenjo-Daro and Haraappa; their remains have proven they are not related to the *Aryans*, who settled the *Punjab and Gangetic Plain*, and were an ancient race of serpent people, who descended from the sky and taught mankind.

The ancient Mayan people of Central America were called "People of the Serpent," the first inhabitants of Yukatan. [8] In the *Book of Numbers*, Moses held up a *Bronzed Serpent* to heal the Israelites. Scripture reads: "And the Lord said to Moses, "Make a fiery serpent, and set it on a pole; and everyone who is bitten, when he sees it, shall live. So Moses made a bronzed serpent and set it on a pole; and if a serpent bit any man, he would look at the bronze serpent and live."[9] Of course, the same Lord sent the original fiery serpents that bit the people; the Israelites began to whine shortly after their escape from Egypt, and many Israelites

---

4   James, 73.

5   Maybe this means he later became Apollo or Zeus?

6   James, 74.

7   Boulay, 47.

8   Boulay, 42, 49.

9   Read Book of Numbers 21:8.

died. Most Christian scholars say the image of the bronzed serpent is a *typology of Jesus Christ*, who forewarned that His angels would rescue us at the end of time — did He not say they will come suddenly from the sky in the Synoptic Gospels?[10]

About the Story

My Epic celebrates Daniel's experiences in Babylon, about what he sensed when he was there, the wisdom he relates to his old friends when he returns home, and the return of *Sky Lord* who rescues the *Sister Woman* in his Divine Chariot, brings her to meet *Father*; they once again return to an Earth in peace. My play is *un devin fantasticque*, that has drawn from the most ancient of religious histories, and molded them together with *Judeo-Christian* scriptures, and also imagined part of my own story being told through a theatrically religious venue. I think I have written a story for which people of all faiths and religions could enjoy, for ancient history and literature scholars, for children, for the entire family. All religions of the earth know about "men" from the sky - no big secret; however, UFO sightings have reportedly increased since 1947 and people want some answers. I do not want people to interpret this play merely on a religious or mystical level, however, for, as an eighteenth-century British Literature student, I can assure everyone that the play is political and open to various interpretations.

On an uncomplicated level, the play is a dramatic, romantic, and sweet story of Daniel, who leaves his woods to visit Babylon and returns to find his friends waiting for him at home. Daniel and the Sister Woman meet Sky Lord, who takes the Sister Woman to meet Father. Sky Lord and the Sister Woman return to earth and to the Forest "to wed in Father's pine grove," and be at peace.

Rocketships in Ancient Babylon

The people of ancient Babylon attempted to build a launch tower for skyborne vehicles. The *Book of Genesis* from the *Hebrew Bible* describes the attempt of the people of Shinar to build a *shem*, or rocketship, to reach father god in the heavens; they were not building a Tower, they were building a launch pad for a rocket. According to *Genesis*, the Lord decided at that point to confuse the language of the people and have them emigrate to different areas of the earth. According to Zecharia Sitchin, "The Bible identifies the place where the attempt to scale the heavens had taken place as Babylon, explaining its Hebrew name Babel as derived from the root 'to confuse.' In fact the original Mesopotamian name, Bab-ili, meant 'Gateway of the Gods,'" a place where the Anunn'aki squabbled over a launch site in 3450 B.C.[11]

---

10   Read Luke: 21:20-33; Matthew 24:28-31 partially reads, "...and he will send out his angels, with a loud trumpet call, and they will gather his elect from the four winds, from one end of heaven to the other."

11   Zecharia Sitchin, *Divine Encounters*: New York: Avon, 1996, 114-115

Recent Literature on Ancient Sky Visitors

I have been most interested of late in some of Zecharia Sitchin's theories in *The Earth Chronicles,* or in books by R.A. Boulay, a former cryptologist from NSA, and by Dr. Arthur David Horn,[12] a physical anthropologist and Yale graduate, that chronicle earth's ancient beginnings in Sumer when the *Anunn'aki*[13], the sons of An or Anu, came to earth; the Anunn'aki's descendants were later referred to in the Old Testament as *Nephilim, the Giants*[14], *Anakim,* and the *Rephaim,* who were all Anunn'aki and human *genetic hybrids.*[15] These "gods" retreated to their spaceships and left mankind and their hybrid offspring to perish in the Flood; they later returned and produced semi-divine offspring called Rephaim—very tall people—to rule earth. Much later on in the *Old Testament,* when Joshua's spies returned from *Canaan,* they related the land of Canaan was the land of *Anakim,* and the spies felt "like grasshoppers" there. Anunn'aki are later referred to in the Hebrew Bible as the *Amal'akites.* In the *Book of Genesis,* Moses and the Israelites fought and mowed down the *Am'alek* at *Reph'idim* with the help of the great *I AM—Yahweh—Jehovah God.*[16]

Ancient Spaceports

The connection between Sitchin's ideas *and The Egyptian Book of the Dead* were also useful in writing my opera. In *Divine Encounters,* Sitchin writes:

> "The subterranean journey inside this sacred mountain of Gilgamesh…is clearly paralleled by the description in The Egyptian Book of the Dead of the pharaoh's subterranean journey…The Pharaoh asked for a shem—a rocketship—with which to ascend to heavenward and join the gods in the eternal abode.…the Sumerian king's and Egyptian Pharaoh's destination

---

12 I am referring to R.A. Boulay's *Flying Serpents and Dragons.* Escondido: The Book Tree, 1999, and Dr. Horn's Humanity 's Extraterrestrial Origins. California: Silberschnur, 1994.

14 Some of the most popular stories in the Old Testaments involve the giants, Og, King of Bashan, and Goliath.

15 Some say these hybrids were the first pharaohs of Egypt. Both the mythical Sphinx and the scriptural cherubim of Ezaekiel are "hybrid" beings combining two to four creatures.

16 Genesis 17:8-13.

17 Sitchin, 158.

18 Abraham went to Egypt during the Bronze Age, when the Age of the Pharaohs had already begun, over one-thousand years before Kings David and Solomon.

12 I am referring to R.A. Boulay's Flying Serpents and Dragons. Escondido: The Book Tree, 1999, and Dr. Horn's Humanity 's Extraterrestrial Origins. California: Silberschnur, 1994.

13 I will use the Semitic spelling here; the ancient Sumerian term for them is Anunna.

14 Some of the most popular stories in the Old Testaments involve the giants, Og, King of Bashan, and Goliath.

15 Some say these hybrids were the first pharaohs of Egypt. Both the mythical Sphinx and the scriptural cherubim of Ezekiel are "hybrid" beings combining two to four creatures.

16 Genesis 17:8-13

was one and the same…the destination was the Spaceport in the Sinai peninsula, where the shems, in their underground silos were." [17]

Sitchin talks of the southernmost point of the *Sinai Peninsula* having been one of the chief Anunn'aki *spaceports*, one of Abraham's destinations[18]; sites of other spaceports were in *Baalbek,* and, of course, *The Temple Mount*, which was the stone landing pad of either Anu orYahweh, millenia before Solomon's Temple.[19] [20] I think mankind has a collective amnesia about its origins and the sacredness of this origin. The Pharaohs in Egypt were anointed by the oil of the sacred crocodile, a direct reference to the blessings of the ancient "reptilian" or "serpent-dragon" gods, allowing one of their "changelings"[21] to rule as King in Egypt. I believe these beings have linguistically descended to us in this reptilian way graphically because of their armored space suits, and their spaceships' ability to laser and destroy; serpent gods, contrary to the *reptilian* designate, are said to be very beautiful beings resembling human kind. I embrace some of Sitchin's ideas—not all—that seem to clarify many of the religious "mysteries" I had been taught were incomprehensible mysteries, which they are not. While I am grounded in the *Jewish* and *Christian* scriptural traditions from religious schools in my youth, I did not feel I had obtained the ultimate truth about man's ancient past. These new ideas in no way diminish what I had originally been taught or believe in, but further enhance my understanding of this planet's unique ancient history, and how very closely we are connected, and yet squabble violently over interpretations of God.

My Intentions for This Book

I have been searching for a written venue to satisfy my many interests—international politics, Middle East studies, British Literature, ancient Sumerian writings and graphics, world religions, the resolution of religious conflicts, poetry, drama, dance, theater, music, archaeology of Ancient History—to merge together a fresh type of verse epic, a *Word Opera.* I have intended this book to be published as a book, a CD, with the hopes that the drama could be eventually recited or chanted as a theatrical piece.

I think artistic interpretations of the piece will vary widely, an intentional move on my part to make the script accessible to people of all cultures and religions, as well as a marketable and profitable venture. The play is written as a two-hour production. I intended the play to be a beautiful story with complex religious and

---

17   Sitchin, 158.

18   Abraham went to Egypt during the Bronze Age, when the Age of the Pharaohs had laready begun, over one-thusand years before King David and Solomon

19   Jerusalem area was the most sacred place on earth before the tribes of Israel were formed.

20   Solomon reigned from 961-925 B.C.

21   A changeling is an offspring of an ancient god or goddess and a human.

linguistic ideas. I want people to come away from theatrical productions with a sense of peace and beauty that currently runs in opposition to the ways things appear, and how people feel today.

Basic Plot

The Hanging Gardens of Babylon tells a story of Daniel, who leaves his Father's Forest to visit Babylon. Daniel receives several visitors in Babylon—the prophet Isaiah, Rabbis, Imams, Jeremiah, Ezekiel, Sumerian women, Moses, Jacob, and Gabriel. **In Part I,** some visitors teach and other visitors listen to Daniel, as he explains his experience in Babylon. Daniel returns to his Forest to be met by his friends and Sister Woman; Daniel shares his experiences in Babylon with them. **In Part II,** Daniel, his friends, and Sister Woman are visited by Sky Lord, who takes Sister Woman to meet the Father, who lives in the sky; the play ends with Sky Lord and Sister Woman's final return to earth to wed in The Forest.

Daniel can be interpreted as the Daniel of the Bible, or he can simply be interpreted as a young man, who ventures away from home, later to recount his findings. The play was written not just on the religious level, so I don't want the religious to feel I am perverting scripture—I have simply written a play. I was raised and educated as a Roman Catholic in Massachusetts; my Grandfather Coulter was an Anglican, who married Margaret Corley, whose Irish Catholic family had been one of the first settlers of Fitchburg in the mid-eighteenth century. I was baptized into the non-instrumental Church of Christ in the mid-1970s in Dublin, Ireland, but have not attended any services of that church since 1980.

I studied Hebrew at a conservative synagogue in Philadelphia for six months; I practiced singing with the Cantor, and the Rabbi allowed me to sing Tenor in their chorus for the High Holy days in the late 1990s, which was a rare privilege. I have enjoyed exploring scripture as my singular avocation into divine mysteries that perked my imagination as a young girl studying God for twelve years in Parochial school and private Catholic girls' academy. My love of religion was interrupted by my love of theater for about ten years, when I lived in Ireland and studied at the Abbey Theatre and at the Gate Theatre, where I acted and worked as Assistant Stage Manager. I appeared on RTE radio and television, played summer stock in New England and performed in three California productions, but I left that objective via other forces for equally interesting pursuits.

Possible Venues and Interpretations of the Play

The play, of course, almost like a *Renaissance or Elizabethan Masque* in a classically political sense, is imagined as a spectacle on a grand stage because of the large cast and chorus. The setting and backgrounds must be vibrant, and drawn according to a similitude of the graphics I have already inserted. The graphics I have currently chosen could be used in the book publication; these graphics are meant to resemble the type of scenic backgrounds I visualize for each scene produced on stage or film. I hear the words chanted in some cases—as when Imams or Cantors chant

The *Greek Chorus*, which I have used throughout, is integral to the movement of scenes, and could also drive the play's production to be staged as a military battle—a type of aerial-ground conflict—there are endless interpretations. I choose words carefully, so the play can be interpreted on many levels, the ultimate objective of L'Art. The choruses are a composite of my study of Irish and English music together with my linguistic choices to invent sounds, and the influence of having attended more than 11 years of piano, dance, and voice in my childhood.

Language of the Play and Cultural Influences

Linguistically, I have purposefully avoided use of articles, unnecessary adjectives, adverbs, and verbs. I hear the language as simple, but not primitive, following a definitive beat that is poetic and yet fresh to the ear, recalling the time when "...the whole earth had one language and few words."[22] I have used the term **E.RIDU**, the ancient *Sumerian* name for the first city on earth, from which the word for Earth originated; and, The Forest setting can be interpreted as a *typology* of **E.DIN**, one of Earth's original spaceports.

This abbreviated style of writing come from my many years of Latin study, my brief Hebrew synagogue studies in Philadelphia, but more strongly is the product of the writing style I learned at the *Central Intelligence Agency,* as part of my training at the *Sherman Kent School of Analysis*; their style was rather terse, in opposition to my more academic style, which is articulated using a few more words. I also studied the Russian language at the Defense Language Institute in Monterey, California, decades before I went to C.I.A. The C.I.A is a unique chapter in my life; I always did love a good mystery.

In terms of *subjective characterization*, I think I am part Daniel and part Sister Woman in the play; Daniel as the "experiencer," and Sister Woman, who loves Sky Lord. I could see Jacob in the wilderness, struggling with the Angel of God; I could hear the approach of Nebu'chard'nez'za from a chorus, but I only heard about his "coming to town," so he never appears as a character. I laid my memory down about my father's woods in Fitchburg, Massachusetts, and went back in my imagination to the smell of pine trees and our brook, to the silence of snow and wind—such peace. In my woods lived the English and Irish with French, Italians, Finns, Greeks, and Native Americans from the region. Some of the Canadian French people in our woods spoke in an interesting dialect, which I have used in parts of the play.

---

22   Read Genesis 11:1.

My French *Aubuchon* family left Dieppe, France, in the early seventeenth century and migrated to the Quebec region of Canada about 1640. I am currently investigating the historical meaning of this move at a rather odd time, one-hundred fifty years before the French Revolution. My French family is one of the original French colonizing families in Canada, a part of the original 15,000. I have always had an interest in the Middle East, and decided to have a bit of linguistic fun with the name "Aubuchon" in the text of the play, and have metamorphisized the name as *Abu'Khan*, which means Son of the Snake, a connection to the ancient Dragon gods spoken of earlier. I had considered using *Abu'chan*, but that name would not have the same linguistic connotation.

My grandfather, John Edward *Coulter* Sr., migrated from Normantown inYorkshire, England, in the late nineteenth century to Fitchburg, Massachusetts; he later served the United States Army as a veteran of the Spanish American War in Cuba. His mother was Sarah Hudson, a direct descendant of Henry Hudson the explorer. I followed my grandfather Coulter's tradition, and served in United States Army Intelligence for a time, and was honorably discharged with the Good Conduct Medal. I believe in the need for having the strongest military on earth to protect and defend against rapid approaches against our own country. I want the reader to understand my cultural heritage in order to understand what I have written; I cannot entirely divorce my cultural, environmental, and religious origins and experiences from the religious aspects of my script.

Musical Intentions

I hear music in the words, I heard the beat throughout the poem, and have utilized some ancient Irish choruses from folk songs that I learned years ago while studying at the *Abbey and Gate Theatres* in Ireland. Other choruses I learned from *old English folk songs,* and with some choruses I just used my *imagination* as a guide in the best *Wordsworthian* tradition.

I would like to hear and see many musical interpretations of the opera. I'd like to hear a symphony behind this piece, a very large orchestra. The types of instruments could vary according to production location. I would like to hear a flourish of trumpets at the beginning and end of Part I and Part Two. I hear many drums, sometimes accompanying the words of individual characters; hear pianos, harps, and strings during scenes in the Forest; hear Bagpipes and harps in the final scene. Music in scenes in Babylon should sound middle-eastern or maybe Chinese. -*Dr. Deborah Coulter-Harris*, Summer, 2005.

Appendix 17

Everyone Loves a Harlot, but Can You trust Her?
By Dr. Deborah M. Coulter-Harris, Philadelphia, 1999

Bernard Mandeville, a Dutch physician who lived in London during the Eighteenth Century, wrote a famous fable entitled *Private Vices, Public Benefits*. In the fable, Mandeville proposes that the profligate and most mischievous people in society actually render economic good for the public, and that a healthy society requires a ration of private vice. He suggests that harlots serve an especially useful function in alleviating the sexual frustrations of powerful men who are scorned by virtuous women and frigid wives. Let's face it, we would rather have our leaders push their bottoms than their nuclear buttons.

World history informs us that there is a long lineage of harlots who have either facilitated the ascent of great leaders, or who have destroyed them. One of the most famous harlots in ancient times was Rahab; she was not only a whore, she was a political collaborator with the revolutionary Joshua against her own king and fellow citizens at Jericho. When Rahab's king sent his men to ask her to inform against the spies, Rahab lied and told the soldiers of Jericho that she didn't know who they were or where they went, but that the soldiers should look for the spies and kill them. Of course Rahab lied to the King and soldiers of Jericho because she had heard of the power of Joshua, and she was afraid that she would perish with the already doomed people and city.

She made Joshua's spies promise that they would save her and all her relatives when they besieged and overthrew the city. She enabled the spies to escape undiscovered and unharmed; she tied a red cord to her window so that Joshua's soldiers would know what one house to leave unharmed when they came to destroy the city. And indeed, Rahab and her house survived the slaughter; afterwards they lived with Joshua and his people for the rest of their lives in prosperity.

Now, I'm not about to propose that the biblical story of Rahab should not be taken seriously; Rahab is certainly a biblical heroine for she did side with the truth, as truth is perceived. However, we do see from Rahab's story that harlots are deceptive wenches, whose only loyalty to political faction rests with the one who wields the most power. Harlots will betray anyone for a bowl of rice. I'm sure that Rahab's immediate thought was how she was going to feed herself and her family if there were no men left in Jericho to service, after Joshua's army slaughtered them all. Most of all, Rahab did not want to die, and so her propensity for self-survival was rewarded.

A really duplicitous and despicable harlot was the woman Delilah. She became lover to Samson, an anointed judge and the strongest man of the ancient world. She betrayed Samson to his Philistine enemies for eleven hundred pieces of silver, as her Philistine friends wanted to destroy the source of Samson's strength. Samson eventually caved into the harlot, and he revealed his secret after she played the old head game, "If you really loved me, you'd tell me all your secrets." Of course, Samson was stupid enough to believe that the harlot really loved him; she only wanted fame and fortune. Samson shared his secret, his hair was cut, he lost his strength, his eyes were cut from his head, and he was sent to prison.

So we see that some harlots only cavort with powerful men to rob them of reputation, to gain intelligence for their enemies, and to collect the riches and fame they will receive from a lascivious public. Of course the commerce involved in such scandals, according to Mandeville's theory, will only booster the economy with book sales, television interviews, etc., a result not entirely disadvantageous for the public economy.

Jezebel was a harlot of another ilk; she was married to the king of Israel and she was a bit of a power-hungry pagan. Jezebel killed all the prophets in the land because they threatened her power. Unfortunately, Jezebel came up against the wrong person when she threatened the life of the great and powerful prophet Elijah because he endangered her political power. Her life ended when her body was thrown into the streets and was eaten by dogs, an event fulfilling Elijah's previous prophecy and curse upon her. So we glean from this story that not all harlots are sexual whores, but some harlots are political whores, harlots for power.

SECTION ONE
Writing the Real World

PART II

READING & WRITING MEMORIES

Preface to Readings

2 July, 2006
Dear Readers,

When I began this book, I did not think of including readings and my commentaries of various writers of the ages. I think this second part of the book could be used a textbook, or simply for popular reading. My choices are somewhat political in nature, so I include favorite political and popular pieces from our past. I also include readings that might be helpful in discussing global trends; I also want to include some of my favorite American and British writers, and include some of my earlier literary analysis. I think training in literary analysis, with close analytical reading—evaluating the possibilities of meanings—is perfect training for future intelligence and business analysts.

I have read many textbooks in my life and engaged in close readings of varied documents: news reports, academic articles, and many books. I could never include all my favorites in this book, as that would fill volumes. I would like to share a few readings that have influenced my life and writing journey, my thinking, and perspective. I am including discussion and writing ideas for instructors and students. I also include my commentary on selected poetry and prose.

As a child, my parents gave me a collection of old books on astronomy and other hard sciences. I remember the feel of the deep-red leather covers, and sitting in my room my head ached from technicalities. I began reading poetry at a very young age. The Sisters of the Presentation in grammar and high schools taught us the great American and English authors and made us memorize and recite many pieces; in high school, the Sisters taught us Latin and we translated many ancient writers. Reading has always been central to my life, and I have pursued many avenues of learning. I hope the reader enjoys the challenges these readings will present; I include questions for reflection or discussion.

Section I

Political Science Readings

1.a. The Clash of Civilizations

by Samuel P. Huntington

*This essay later became a book by the same name. Students should enjoy this essay, as it **predicts a possible global future based upon cultural and religious divides.** Huntington may be right, but I think we might become so globalized that the probability we are going to have a one-world order and world religion ranks among possibilities—how else will we survive? I am including writing and discussion suggestions.*

In-class Writing and Team Exercise Response to Huntington's Essay

WRITING ALONE (30 minutes) *1 page*

Please write a 1 to 2 page essay response to the reading, *The Clash of Civilizations.* Answer the following questions, but write the assignment in essay form:

1.   What is Huntington's thesis?

2.   What is his argument?

3.   Talk about at least three of the author's main points that support his thesis.
     ①similar civs. =war ;②after WWII things manifested & got worse,

4.   Does Huntington offer any solutions to the problem he discusses? What does he forecast for the future?

5.   Does the author call upon readers to take some action? If so, please identify these actions?

6.   Propose a resolution to one of the conflicts that Huntington mentions in his essay, using Divergent/Convergent thinking process.

WORKING IN TEAMS (45 minutes)

Using one of the critical thinking skills you have recently learned in this course—either the decision event tree or divergent/convergent thinking—please propose a solution to one of the conflicts/problems that Huntington identifies in his essay.

Samuel P. Huntington, "The Clash of Civilizations?" Foreign Affairs *Summer 1993, 72/3.*

SAMUEL P. HUNTINGTON is the Eaton Professor of the Science of Government and Director of the John M. Olin Institute for Strategic Studies at Harvard University. This article is the product of the Olin Institute's project on "The Changing Security Environment and American National Interests."

Sections:

i.   **The Next Pattern of Conflict**

ii.   **The Nature of Civilizations**

iii.   **Why Civilizations Will Clash**

iv.   **The Fault Lines Between Civilizations**

v.   **Civilization Rallying**

I. The Next Pattern of Conflict

WORLD POLITICS IS entering a new phase, and intellectuals have not hesitated to proliferate visions of what it will be — the end of history, the return of traditional rivalries between nation states, and the decline of the nation state from the conflicting pulls of tribalism and globalism, among others. Each of these visions catches aspects of the emerging reality. Yet they all miss a crucial, indeed a central, aspect of what global politics is likely to be in the coming years.

It is my hypothesis that the fundamental source of conflict in this new world will not be primarily ideological or primarily economic. The great divisions among humankind and the dominating source of conflict will be cultural. Nation states will remain the most powerful actors in world affairs, but the principal conflicts of global politics will occur between nations and groups of different civilizations. The clash of civilizations will be the battle lines of the future.

Conflict between civilizations will be the latest phase of the evolution of conflict in the modern world. For a century and a half after the emergence of the modern international system of the Peace of Westphalia, the conflicts of the Western world were largely among princes — emperors, absolute monarchs and constitutional monarchs attempting to expand their bureaucracies, their armies, their mercantilist economic strength and, most important, the territory they ruled. In the process they created nation states, and beginning with the French Revolution the principal lines of conflict were between nations rather than princes. In 1793, as R. R. Palmer put it, "The wars of kings were over; the ward of peoples had begun." This nineteenth-century pattern lasted until the end of World War I. Then, as a result of the Russian Revolution and the reaction against it, the conflict of nations yielded to the conflict of ideologies, first among communism, fascism-Nazism and liberal democracy, and then between communism and liberal democracy. During the Cold War, this latter conflict became embodied in the struggle between the two superpowers, neither of which was a nation state in the classical European sense and each of which defined its identity in terms of ideology.

These conflicts between princes, nation states and ideologies were primarily conflicts within Western civilization, "Western civil wars," as William Lind has labeled them. This was as true of the Cold War as it was of the world wars and the earlier wars of the seventeenth, eighteenth and nineteenth centuries. With the end of the Cold War, international politics moves out of its Western phase, and its center-piece becomes the interaction between the West and non-Western civilizations and among non-Western civilizations. In the politics of civilizations, the people and governments of non-Western civilizations no longer remain the objects of history as targets of Western colonialism but join the West as movers and shapers of history.

II. The Nature of Civilizations

DURING THE COLD WAR the world was divided into the First, Second and Third Worlds. Those divisions are no longer relevant. It is far more meaningful now to group countries not in terms of their political or economic systems or in terms of their level of economic development but rather in terms of their culture and civilization.

What do we mean when we talk of a civilization? A civilization is a cultural entity. Villages, regions, ethnic groups, nationalities, religious groups, all have distinct cultures at different levels of cultural heterogeneity. The culture of a village in southern Italy may be different from that of a village in northern Italy, but both will share in a common Italian culture that distinguishes them from German villages. European communities, in turn, will share cultural features that distinguish them from Arab or Chinese communities. Arabs, Chinese and Westerners, however, are not part of any broader cultural entity. They constitute civilizations. A civilization is thus the highest cultural grouping of people and the broadest level of cultural identity people have short of that which distinguishes humans from other species. It is defined both by common objective elements, such as language, history, religion, customs, institutions, and by the subjective self-identification of people. People have levels of identity: a resident of Rome may define himself with varying degrees of intensity as a Roman, an Italian, a Catholic, a Christian, a European, a Westerner. The civilization to which he belongs is the broadest level of identification with which he intensely identifies. People can and do redefine their identities and, as a result, the composition and boundaries of civilizations change.

Civilizations may involve a large number of people, as with China ("a civilization pretending to be a state," as Lucian Pye put it), or a very small number of people, such as the Anglophone Caribbean. A civilization may include several nation states, as is the case with Western, Latin American and Arab civilizations, or only one, as is the case with Japanese civilization. Civilizations obviously blend and overlap, and may include subcivilizations. Western civilization has two major variants, European and North American, and Islam has its Arab, Turkic and Malay subdivisions. Civilizations are nonetheless meaningful entities, and while the lines between them are seldom sharp, they are real. Civilizations are dynamic; they rise and fall; they divide and merge. And, as any student of history knows, civilizations disappear and are buried in the sands of time.

Westerners tend to think of nation states as the principal actors in global affairs. They have been that, however, for only a few centuries. The broader reaches of human history have been the history of civilizations. In A Study of History, Arnold Toynbee identified 21 major civilizations; only six of them exist in the contemporary world.

III. Why Civilizations will Clash

CIVILIZATION IDENTITY will be increasingly important in the future, and the world will be shaped in large measure by the interactions among seven or eight major civilizations. These include Western, Confucian, Japanese, Islamic, Hindu, Slavic-Orthodox, Latin American and possibly African civilization. The most important conflicts of the future will occur along the cultural fault lines separating these civilizations from one another.

Why will this be the case?

First, differences among civilizations are not only real; they are basic. Civilizations are differentiated from each other by history, language, culture, tradition and, most important, religion. The people of different civilizations have different views on the relations between God and man, the individual and the group, the citizen and the state, parents and children, husband and wife, as well as differing views of the relative importance of rights and responsibilities, liberty and authority, equality and hierarchy. These differences are the product of centuries. They will not soon disappear. They are far more fundamental than differences among political ideologies and political regimes. Differences do not necessarily mean conflict, and conflict does not necessarily mean violence. Over the centuries, however, differences among civilizations have generated the most prolonged and the most violent conflicts.

Second, the world is becoming a smaller place. The interactions between peoples of different civilizations are increasings; these increasing interactions intensify civilization consciousness and awareness of differences between civilizations and commonalities within civilizations. North African immigration to France generates hostility among Frenchmen and at the same time increased receptivity to immigration by "good" European Catholic Poles. Americans react far more negatively to Japanese investment than to larger investments from Canada and European countries. Similarly, as Donald Horowitz has pointed out, "An Ibo may be . . . an Owerri Ibo or an Onitsha Ibo in what was the Eastern region of Nigeria. In Lagos, he is simply an Ibo. In London, he is a Nigerian. In New York, he is an African." The interactions among peoples of different civilizations enhance the civilization-consciousness of people that, in turn, invigorates differences and animosities stretching or thought to stretch back deep into history.

Third, the processes of economic modernization and social change throughout the world are separating people from longstanding local identities. They also weaken the nation state as a source of identity. In much of the world religion has moved in to fill this gap, often in the form of movements that are labeled "fundamentalist." Such movements are found in Western Christianity, Judaism, Buddhism and Hinduism, as well as in Islam. In most countries and most religions the people active in fundamentalist movements are young, college-educated, middle-class technicians, professionals and business persons. The "unsecularization of the world," George Weigel has remarked, "is one of the dominant social factors of life in the late twentieth century." The revival of religion, "la revanche de Dieu," as Gilles Kepel labeled it, provides a basis for identity and commitment that transcends national boundaries and unites civilizations.

Fourth, the growth of civilization-consciousness is enhanced by the dual role of the West. On the one hand, the West is at a peak of power. At the same time, however, and perhaps as a result, a return to the roots phenomenon is occurring among non-Western civilizations. Increasingly one hears references to trends toward a turning inward and "Asianization" in Japan, the end of the Nehru legacy and the "Hinduization" of India, the failure of Western ideas of socialism and nationalism and hence "re-Islamization" of the Middle East, and now a debate over Westernization versus Russianization in Boris Yeltsin's country. A West at the peak of its power confronts non-Wests that increasingly have the desire, the will and the resources to shape the world in non-Western ways.

In the past, the elites of non-Western societies were usually the people who were most involved with the West, had been educated at Oxford, the Sorbonne or Sandhurst, and had absorbed Western attitudes and values. At the same time, the populace in non-Western countries often remained deeply imbued with the indigenous culture. Now, however, these relationships are being reversed. A de-Westernization and indigenization of elites is occurring in many non-Western countries at the same time that Western, usually American, cultures, styles and habits become more popular among the mass of the people.

Fifth, cultural characteristics and differences are less mutable and hence less easily compromised and resolved than political and economic ones. In the former Soviet Union, communists can become democrats, the rich can become poor and the poor rich, but Russians cannot become Estonians and Azeris cannot become Armenians. In class and ideological conflicts, the key question was "Which side are you on?" and people could and did choose sides and change sides. In conflicts between civilizations, the question is "What are you?" That is a given that cannot be changed. And as we know, from Bosnia to the Caucasus to the Sudan, the wrong answer to that question can mean a bullet in the head. Even more than ethnicity, religion discriminates sharply and exclusively among people. A person can be half-French and half-Arab and simultaneously even a citizen of two countries. It is more difficult to be half-Catholic and half-Muslim.

Finally, economic regionalism is increasing. The proportions of total trade that are intraregional rose between 1980 and 1989 from 51 percent to 59 percent in Europe, 33 percent to 37 percent in East Asia, and 32 percent to 36 percent in North America. The importance of regional economic blocs is likely to continue to increase in the future. On the one hand, successful economic regionalism will reinforce civilization-consciousness. On the other hand, economic regionalism may succeed only when it is rooted in a common civilization. The European Community rests on the shared foundation of European culture and Western Christianity. The success of the North American Free Trade Area depends on the convergence now underway of Mexican, Canadian and American cultures. Japan, in contrast, faces difficulties in creating a comparable economic entity in East Asia because Japan is a society and civilization unique to itself. However strong the trade and investment links Japan may develop with other East Asian countries, its cultural differences with those countries inhibit and perhaps preclude its promoting regional economic integration like that in Europe and North America.

Common culture, in contrast, is clearly facilitating the rapid expansion of the economic relations between the People's Republic of China and Hong Kong, Taiwan, Singapore and the overseas Chinese communities in other Asian countries. With the Cold War over, cultural commonalities increasingly overcome ideological differences, and mainland China and Taiwan move closer together. If cultural commonality is a prerequisite for economic integration, the principal East Asian economic bloc of the future is likely to be centered on China. This bloc is, in fact, already coming into existence. As Murray Weidenbaum has observed,

Despite the current Japanese dominance of the region, the Chinese-based economy of Asia is rapidly emerging as a new epicenter for industry, commerce and finance. This strategic area contains substantial amounts of technology and manufacturing capability (Taiwan), outstanding entrepreneurial, marketing and services acumen (Hong Kong), a fine communications network (Singapore), a tremendous pool of financial capital (all three), and very large endowments of land, resources and labor (mainland China). . . . From Guangzhou to Singapore, from Kuala Lumpur to Manila, this influential network — often based on extensions of the traditional clans — has been described as the backbone of the East Asian economy. (1)

Culture and religion also form the basis of the Economic Cooperation Organization, which brings together ten non-Arab Muslim countries: Iran, Pakistan, Turkey, Azerbaijan, Kazakhstan, Kyrgyzstan, Turkmenistan, Tadjikistan, Uzbekistan and Afghanistan. One impetus to the revival and expansion of this organization, founded originally in the 1960s by Turkey, Pakistan and Iran, is the realization by the leaders of several of these countries that they had no chance of admission to the European Community. Similarly, Caricom, the Central American Common Market and Mercosur rest on common cultural foundations. Efforts to build a broader Caribbean-Central American economic entity bridging the Anglo-Latin divide, however, have to date failed.

As people define their identity in ethnic and religious terms, they are likely to see an "us" versus "them" relation existing between themselves and people of different ethnicity or religion. The end of ideologically defined states in Eastern Europe and the former Soviet Union permits traditional ethnic identities and animosities to come to the fore. Differences in culture and religion create differences over policy issues, ranging from human rights to immigration to trade and commerce to the environment. Geographical propinquity gives rise to conflicting territorial claims from Bosnia to Mindanao. Most important, the efforts of the West to promote its values of democracy and liberalism to universal values, to maintain its military predominance and to advance its economic interests engender countering responses from other civilizations. Decreasingly able to mobilize support and form coalitions on the basis of ideology, governments and groups will increasingly attempt to mobilize support by appealing to common religion and civilization identity.

The clash of civilizations thus occurs at two levels. At the micro-level, adjacent groups along the fault lines between civilizations struggle, often violently, over the control of territory and each other. At the macro-level, states from different civilizations compete for relative military and economic power, struggle over the control of international institutions and third parties, and competitively promote their particular political and religious values.

IV. *The Fault Lines Between Civilizations*

THE FAULT LINES between civilizations are replacing the political and ideological boundaries of the Cold War as the flash points for crisis and bloodshed. The Cold War began when the Iron Curtain divided Europe politically and ideologically. The Cold War ended with the end of the Iron Curtain. As the ideological division of Europe has disappeared, the cultural division of Europe between Western Christianity, on the one hand, and Orthodox Christianity and Islam, on the other, has reemerged. The most significant dividing line in Europe, as William Wallace has suggested, may well be the eastern boundary of Western Christianity in the year 1500. This line runs along what are now the boundaries between Finland and Russia and between the Baltic states and Russia, cuts through Belarus and Ukraine separating the more Catholic western Ukraine from Orthodox eastern Ukraine, swings westward separating Transylvania from the rest of Romania, and then goes through Yugoslavia almost exactly along the line now separating Croatia and Slovenia from the rest of Yugoslavia. In the Balkans this line, of course, coincides with the historic boundary between the Hapsburg and Ottoman empires. The peoples to the north and west of this line are Protestant or Catholic; they shared the common experiences of European history — feudalism, the Renaissance, the Reformation, the Enlightenment, the French Revolution, the Industrial Revolution; they are generally economically better off than the peoples to the east; and they may now look forward to increasing involvement in a common European economy and to the consolidation of democratic political systems. The peoples to the east and south of this line are Orthodox or Muslim; they historically belonged to the Ottoman or Tsarist empires and were only lightly touched by the shaping events in the rest of Europe; they are generally less advanced economically; they seem much less likely to develop stable democratic political systems. The Velvet Curtain of culture has replaced the Iron Curtain of ideology as the most significant dividing line in Europe. As the events in Yugoslavia show, it is not only a line of difference; it is also at times a line of bloody conflict.

Conflict along the fault line between Western and Islamic civilizations has been going on for 1,300 years. After the founding of Islam, the Arab and Moorish surge west and north only ended at Tours in 732. From the eleventh to the thirteenth century the Crusaders attempted with temporary success to bring Christianity and Christian rule to the Holy Land. From the fourteenth to the seventeenth century, the Ottoman Turks reversed the balance, extended their sway over the Middle East and the Balkans, captured Constantinople, and twice laid siege to Vienna. In the nineteenth and early twentieth centuries at Ottoman power declined Britain, France, and Italy established Western control over most of North Africa and the Middle East.

After World War II, the West, in turn, began to retreat; the colonial empires disappeared; first Arab nationalism and then Islamic fundamentalism manifested themselves; the West became heavily dependent on the Persian Gulf countries for its energy; the oil-rich Muslim countries became money-rich and, when they wished to, weapons-rich. Several wars occurred between Arabs and Israel (created by the West). France fought a bloody and ruthless war in Algeria for most of the 1950s; British and French forces invaded Egypt in 1956; American forces returned to Lebanon, attacked Libya, and engaged in various military encounters with Iran; Arab and Islamic terrorists, supported by at least three Middle Eastern governments, employed the weapon of the weak and bombed Western planes and installations and seized Western hostages. This warfare between Arabs and the West culminated in 1990, when the United States sent a massive army to the Persian Gulf to defend some Arab countries against aggression by another. In its aftermath NATO planning is increasingly directed to potential threats and instability along its "southern tier."

This centuries-old military interaction between the West and Islam is unlikely to decline. It could become more virulent. The Gulf War left some Arabs feeling proud that Saddam Hussein had attacked Israel and stood up to the West. It also left many feeling humiliated and resentful of the West's military presence in the Persian Gulf, the West's overwhelming military dominance, and their apparent inability to shape their own destiny. Many Arab countries, in addition to the oil exporters, are reaching levels of economic and social development where autocratic forms of government become inappropriate and efforts to introduce democracy become stronger. Some openings in Arab political systems have already occurred.

The principal beneficiaries of these openings have been Islamist movements. In the Arab world, in short, Western democracy strengthens anti-Western political forces. This may be a passing phenomenon, but it surely complicates relations between Islamic countries and the West.

Those relations are also complicated by demography. The spectacular population growth in Arab countries, particularly in North Africa, has led to increased migration to Western Europe. The movement within Western Europe toward minimizing internal boundaries has sharpened political sensitivities with respect to this development. In Italy, France and Germany, racism is increasingly open, and political reactions and violence against Arab and Turkish migrants have become more intense and more widespread since 1990.

On both sides the interaction between Islam and the West is seen as a clash of civilizations. The West's "next confrontation," observes M. J. Akbar, an Indian Muslim author, "is definitely going to come from the Muslim world. It is in the sweep of the Islamic nations from the Meghreb to Pakistan that the struggle for a new world order will begin." Bernard Lewis comes to a regular conclusion:

> "We are facing a need and a movement far transcending the level of issues and policies and the governments that pursue them. This is no less than a clash of civilizations — the perhaps irrational but surely historic reaction of an ancient rival against our Judeo-Christian heritage, our secular present, and the worldwide expansion of both. (2)

Historically, the other great antagonistic interaction of Arab Islamic civilization has been with the pagan, animist, and now increasingly Christian black peoples to the south. In the past, this antagonism was epitomized in the image of Arab slave dealers and black slaves. It has been reflected in the on-going civil war in the Sudan between Arabs and blacks, the fighting in Chad between Libyan-supported insurgents and the government, the tensions between Orthodox Christians and Muslims in the Horn of Africa, and the political conflicts, recurring riots and communal violence between Muslims and Christians in Nigeria. The modernization of Africa and the spread of Christianity in Nigeria. The modernization of Africa and the spread of Christianity are likely to enhance the probability of violence along this fault line. Symptomatic of the intensification of this conflict was the Pope John Paul II's speech in Khartoum in February 1993 attacking the actions of the Sudan's Islamist government against the Christian minority there.

On the northern border of Islam, conflict has increasingly erupted between Orthodox and Muslim peoples, including the carnage of Bosnia and Sarajevo, the simmering violence between Serb and Albanian, the tenuous relation between Bulgarians and their Turkish minority, the violence between Ossetians and Ingush, the unremitting slaughter of each other by Armenians and Azeris, the tense relations between Russians and Muslims in Central Asia, and the deployment of Russian troops to protect Russian interests in the Caucasus and Central Asia. Religion reinforces the revival of ethnic identities and restimulates Russian fears about the security of their southern borders. This concern is well captured by Archie Roosevelt:

Much of Russian history concerns the struggle between Slavs and the Turkish peoples on their borders, which dates back to the foundation of the Russian state more than a thousand years ago. In the Slavs' millennium-long confrontation with their eastern neighbors lies the key to an understanding not only of Russian history, but Russian character. To under Russian realities today one has to have a concept of the great Turkic ethnic group that has preoccupied Russians through the centuries. (3)

The conflict of civilizations is deeply rooted elsewhere in Asia. The historic clash between Muslim and Hindu in the subcontinent manifests itself now not only is the rivalry between Pakistan and India but also in intensifying religious strife within India between increasingly militant Hindu groups and India's substantial Muslim minority. The destruction of the Ayodhya mosque in December 1992 brought to the fore the issue of whether India will remain a secular democratic state or become a Hindu one. In East Asia, China has outstanding territorial disputes with most of its neighbors. It has pursued a ruthless policy toward the Buddhist people of Tibet, and it is pursuing an increasingly ruthless policy toward its Turkic-Muslim minority. With the Cold War over, the underlying differences between China and the United States have reasserted themselves in areas such as human rights, trade and weapons proliferation. These differences are unlikely to moderate. A "new cold war," Deng Xaioping reportedly asserted in 1991, is under way between China and America.

The same phrase has been applied to the increasingly difficult relations between Japan and the United States. Here cultural difference exacerbates economic conflict. People on each side allege racism on the other, but at least on the American side the antipathies are not racial but cultural. The basic values, attitudes, behavioral patterns of the two societies could hardly be more different. The economic issues between the United States and Europe are no less serious than those between the United States and Japan, but they do not have thesame political salience and emotional intensity because the differences between American culture and European culture are so much less than those between American civilization and Japanese civilization.

The interactions between civilizations vary greatly in the extent to which they are likely to be characterized by violence. Economic competition clearly predominates between the American and European subcivilizations of the West and between both of them and Japan. On the Eurasian continent, however, the proliferation of ethnic conflict, epitomized at the extreme in "ethnic cleansing," has not been totally random. It has been most frequent and most violent between groups belonging to different civilizations. In Eurasia the great historic fault lines between civilizations are once more aflame. This is particularly true along the boundaries of the crescent-shaped Islamic bloc of nations from the bulge of Africa to central Asia. Violence also occurs between Muslims, on the one hand, and Orthodox Serbs in the Balkans, Jews in Israel, Hindus in India, Buddhists in Burma and Catholics in the Philippines. Islam has bloody borders.

V. Civilization Rallying

The kin-country syndrome groups or states belonging to one civilization that become involved in war with people from a different civilization naturally try to rally support from other members of their own civilization. As the post-Cold War world evolves, civilization commonality, what H. D. S. Greenway has termed the "kin-country" syndrome, is replacing political ideology and traditional balance of power considerations as the principal basis for cooperation and coalitions. It can be seen gradually emerging in the post-Cold War conflicts in the Persian Gulf, the Caucasus and Bosnia. None of these was a full-scale war between civilizations, but each involved some elements of civilization rallying, which seemed to become more important as the conflict continued and which may provide a foretaste of the future.

First, in the Gulf War one Arab state invaded another and then fought a coalition of Arab, Western and other states. While only a few Muslim governments overtly supported Saddam Hussein, many Arab elites privately cheered him on, and he was highly popular among large sections of the Arab publics. Islamic fundamentalist movements universally supported Iraq rather than the Western-backed governments of Kuwait and Saudi Arabia. Forswearing Arab nationalism, Saddam Hussein explicitly invoked an Islamic appeal. He and his supporters attempted to define the war as a war between civilizations. "It is not the world against Iraq," as Safar Al-Hawali, dean of Islamic Studies at the Umm Al-Qura University in Mecca, put it in a widely circulated tape. "It is the West against Islam." Ignoring the rivalry between Iran and Iraq, the chief Iranian religious leader, Ayatollah Ali Khamenei, called for a holy war against the West: "The struggle against American aggression, greed, plans and policies will be counted as a jahad, and anybody who is killed on that path is a martyr.""This is a war," King Hussein of Jordan argued, "against all Arabs and all Muslims and not against Iraq alone."

The rallying of substantial sections of Arab elites and publics behind Saddam Hussein called those Arab governments in the anti-Iraq coalition to moderate their activities and temper their public statements. Arab governments opposed or distanced themselves from subsequent Western efforts to apply pressure on Iraq, including enforcement of a no-fly zone in the summer of 1992 and the bombing of Iraq in January 1993. The Western-Soviet-Turkish-Arab anti-Iraq coalition of 1990 had by 1993 become a coalition of almost only the West and Kuwait against Iraq.

Muslims contrasted Western actions against Iraq with the West's failure to protect Bosnians against Serbs and to impose sanctions on Israel for violating U.N. resolutions. The West, they allege, was using a double standard. A world of clashing civilizations, however, is inevitably a world of double standards: people apply one standard to their kin-countries and a different standard to others.

Second, the kin-country syndrome also appeared in conflicts in the former Soviet Union. Armenian military successes in 1992 and 1993 stimulated Turkey to become increasingly supportive of its religious, ethnic and linguistic brethren in Azerbaijan. "We have a Turkish nation feeling the same sentiments as the Azerbaijanis," said one Turkish official in 1992. "We are under pressure. Our newspapers are full of the photos of atrocities and are asking us if we are still serious about pursuing our neutral policy. Maybe we should show Armenia that there's a big Turkey in the region." President Turgut Ozal agreed, remarking that Turkey should at least "scare the Armenians a little bit." Turkey, Ozal threatened again in 1993, would "show its fangs." Turkey Air Force jets flew reconnaissance flights along the Armenian border; Turkey suspended food shipments and air flights to Armenia; and Turkey and Iran announced they would not accept dismemberment of Azerbaijan. In the last years of its existence, the Soviet government supported Azerbaijan because its government was dominated by former communists. With the end of the Soviet Union, however, political considerations gave way to religious ones. Russian troops fought on the Side of the Armenians, and Azerbaijan accused the "Russian government of turning 180 degrees" toward support for Christian Armenia.

Third, with respect to the fighting in the former Yugoslavia, Western publics manifested sympathy and support for the Bosnian Muslims and the horrors they suffered at the hands of the Serbs. Relatively little concern was expressed, however, over Croatian attacks on Muslims and participation in the dismemberment of Bosnia-Herzegovina. In the early stages of the Yugoslav breakup, Germany, in an unusual display of diplomatic initiative and muscle, induced the other 11 members of the European Community to follow its lead in recognizing Slovenia and Croatia. As a result of the pope's determination to provide strong backing to the two Catholic countries, the Vatican extended recognition even before the Community did. The United States followed the European lead. Thus the leading actors in Western civilization rallied behind its coreligionists. Subsequently Croatia was reported to be receiving substantial quantities of arms from Central European and other Western countries. Boris Yeltsin's government, on the other hand, attempted to pursue a middle course that would be sympathetic to the Orthodox Serbs but not alienate Russia from the West. Russian conservative and nationalist groups, however, including many legislators, attacked the government for not being more forthcoming in its support for the Serbs. By early 1993 several hundred Russians apparently were serving with the Serbian forces, and reports circulated of Russian arms being supplied to Serbia.

Islamic governments and groups, on the other hand, castigated the West for not coming to the defense of the Bosnians. Iranian leaders urged Muslims from all countries to provide help to Bosnia; in violation of the U.N. arms embargo, Iran supplied weapons and men for the Bosnians; Iranian-supported Lebanese groups sent guerrillas to train and organize the Bosnian forces.

In 1993 up to 4,000 Muslims from over two dozen Islamic countries were reported to be fighting in Bosnia. The governments of Saudi Arabia and other countries felt under increasing pressure from fundamentalist groups in their own societies to provide more vigorous support for the Bosnians. By the end of 1992, Saudi Arabia had reportedly supplied substantial funding for weapons and supplies for the Bosnians, which significantly increased their military capabilities vis-a-vis the Serbs.

In the 1930s the Spanish Civil War provoked intervention from countries that politically were fascist, communist and democratic. In the 1990s the Yugoslav conflict is provoking intervention from countries that are Muslim, Orthodox and Western Christian. The parallel has not gone unnoticed. "The war in Bosnia-Herzegovina has become the emotional equivalent of the fight against fascism in the Spanish Civil War," one Saudi editor observed. "Those who died there are regarded as martyrs who tried to save their fellow Muslims."

Conflicts and violence will also occur between states and groups within the same civilization. Such conflicts, however, are likely to be less intense and less likely to expand than conflicts between civilizations. Common membership in a civilization reduces the probability of violence in situations where it might otherwise occur. In 1991 and 1992 many people were alarmed by the possibility of violent conflict between Russia and Ukraine over territory, particularly Crimea, the Black Sea fleet, nuclear weapons and economic issues. If civilization is what counts, however, the likelihood of violence between Ukrainians and Russians should be low. They are two Slavic, primarily Orthodox peoples who have had close relationships with each other for centuries. As of early 1993, despite all the reasons for conflict, the leaders of the two countries were effectively negotiating and defusing the issues between the two countries. While there has been serious fighting between Muslims and Christians elsewhere in the former Soviet Union and much tension and some fighting between Western and Orthodox Christians in the Baltic states, there has been virtually no violence between Russians and Ukrainians.

Civilization rallying to date has been limited, but it has been growing, and it clearly has the potential to spread much further. As the conflicts in the Persian Gulf, the Caucasus and Bosnia continued, the positions of nations and the cleavages between them increasingly were along civilizational lines. Populist politicians, religious leaders and the media have found it a potential means of arousing mass support and of pressuring hesitant governments. In the coming years, the local conflicts most likely to escalate into major wars will be those, as in Bosnia and the

Caucasus, along the fault lines between civilizations. The next world war, if there is one, will be a war between civilizations.

VI. The West Versus the Rest

The west is now at an extraordinary peak of power in relation to other civilizations. In superpower opponent has disappeared from the map. Military conflict among Western states is unthinkable, and Western military power is unrivaled. Apart from Japan, the West faces no economic challenge. It dominates international economic institutions. Global political and security issues are effectively settled by a directorate of the United States, Britain and France, world economic issues by a directorate of the United States, Germany and Japan, all of which maintain extraordinarily close relations with each other to the exclusion of lesser and largely non-Western countries. Decisions made at the U.N. Security Council or in the International Monetary Fund that reflect the interests of the West are presented to the world as reflecting the desires of the world community. The very phrase "the world community" has become the euphemistic collective noun (replacing "the Free World") to give global legitimacy to actions reflecting the interests of the United States and other Western powers. (4) Through the IMF and other international economic institutions, the West promotes its economic interests and imposes on other nations the economic policies it thinks appropriate. In any poll of non-Western peoples, the IMF undoubtedly would win the support of finance ministers and a few others, but get an overwhelmingly unfavorable rating from just about everyone else, who would agree with Georgy Arbatov's characterization of IMF officials as "neo-Bolsheviks who love expropriating other people's money, imposing undemocratic and alien rules of economic and political conduct and stifling economic freedom."

Western domination of the U.N. Security Council and its decisions, tempered only by occasional abstention by China, produced U.N. legitimation of the West's use of force to drive Iraq out of Kuwait and its elimination of Iraq's sophisticated weapons and capacity to produce such weapons. It also produced the quite unprecedented action by the United States, Britain and France in getting the Security Council to demand that Libya hand over the Pan Am 103 bombing suspects and then to impose sanctions when Libya refused. After defeating the largest Arab army, the West did not hesistate to throw its weight around in the Arab world. The West in effect is using international institutions, military power and economic resources to run the world in ways that will maintain Western predominance, protect Western interests and promote Western political and economic values.

That at least is the way in which non-Westerners see the new world, and there is a significant element of truth in their view. Differences in power and struggles for military, economic and institutional power are thus one source of conflict between the West and other civilizations. Differences in culture, that is basic values and beliefs, are a second source of conflict. V. S. Naipaul has argued that Western civilization is the "universal civilization" that "fits all men." At a superficial level much of Western culture has indeed permeated the rest of the world. At a more basic level, however, Western concepts differ fundamentally from those prevalent in other civilizations. Western ideas of individualism, liberalism, constitutionalism, human rights, equality, liberty, the rule of law, democracy, free markets, the separation of church and state, often have little resonance in Islamic, Confucian, Japanese, Hindu, Buddhist or Orthodox cultures. Western efforts to propagate each ideas produce instead a reaction against "human rights imperialism" and a reaffirmation of indigenous values, as can be seen in the support for religious fundamentalism by the younger generation in non-Western cultures. The very notion that there could be a "universal civilization" is a Western idea, directly at odds with the particularism of most Asian societies and their emphasis on what distinguishes one people from another. Indeed, the author of a review of 100 comparative studies of values in different societies concluded that "the values that are most important in the West are least important worldwide." (5) In the political realm, of course, these differences are most manifest in the efforts of the United States and other Western powers to induce other peoples to adopt Western ideas concerning democracy and human rights. Modern democratic government originated in the West. When it has developed colonialism or imposition.

The central axis of world politics in the future is likely to be, in Kishore Mahbubani's phrase, the conflict between "the West and the Rest" and the responses of non-Western civilizations to Western power and values. (6) Those responses generally take one or a combination of three forms. At one extreme, non-Western states can, like Burma and North Korea, attempt to pursue a course of isolation, to insulate their societies from penetration or "corruption" by the West, and, in effect, to opt out of participation in the Western-dominated global community. The costs of this course, however, are high, and few states have pursued it exclusively. A second alternative, the equivalent of "band-wagoning" in international relations theory, is to attempt to join the West and accept its values and institutions. The third alternative is to attempt to "balance" the West by developing economic and military power and cooperating with other non-Western societies against the West, while preserving indigenous values and institutions; in short, to modernize but not to Westernize.

VII. The Torn Countries

In the future, as people differentiate themselves by civilization, countries with large numbers of people of different civilizations, such as the Soviet Union and Yugoslavia, are candidates for dismemberment. Some other countries have a fair degree of cultural homogeneity but are divided over whether their society belongs to one civilization or another. These are town countries. Their leaders typically wish to pursue a bandwagoning strategy and to make theirc ountries members of the West, but the history, culture and traditions of their countries are non-Western. The most obvious and prototypical torn country is Turkey. The late twentieth-century leaders of Turkey have followed in the Attaturk tradition and defined Turkey as a modern, secular, Western nation state. They allied Turkey with the West in NATO and in the Gulf War; they applied for membership in the European Community. At the same time, however, elements in Turkish society have supported an Islamic revival and have argued that Turkey is basically a Middle Eastern Muslim society. In addition, while the elite of Turkey has defined Turkey as a Western society, the elite of the West refuses to accept Turkey and such. Turkey will not become a member of the European Community, and the real reason, as President Ozal said, "is that we are Muslim and they are Christian and they don't say that." Having rejected Mecca, and then being rejected by Brussels, where does Turkey look? Tashkent may be the answer. The end of the Soviet Union gives Turkey the opportunity to become the leader of a revived Turkic civilization involving seven countries from the borders of Greece to those of China. Encouraged by the West, Turkey is making strenuous efforts to carve out this new identity for itself.

During the past decade Mexico has assumed a position somewhat similar to that of Turkey. Just as Turkey abandoned its historic opposition to Europe and attempted to join Europe, Mexico has stopped defining itself by its opposition to the United States and is instead attempting to imitate the United States and to join it in the North American Free Trade Area. Mexican leaders are engaged in the great task of redefining Mexican identity and have introduced fundamental economic reforms that eventually will lead to fundamental political change. In 1991 a top adviser to President Carlos Salinas de Gortari described at length tome all the changes the Salinas government was making. When he finished, I remarked: "That's most impressive. It seems to me that basically you want to change Mexico from a Latin American country into a North American country." He looked at me with surprise and exclaimed: "Exactly! That's precisely what we are trying to do, but of course we could never say so publicly." As his remark indicates, in Mexico as in Turkey, significant elements in society resist the redefinition of their country's identity. In Turkey, European-oriented leaders have to make gestures to Islam (Ozal's pilgrimage to Mecca); so also Mexico's North American-oriented leaders have to make gestures to those who hold Mexico to be a Latin American country (Salinas' Ibero-American Guadalajara summit).

Historically Turkey has been the most profoundly torn country. For the United States, Mexico is the most immediate torn country. Globally the most important torn country is Russia. The question of whether Russia is part of the West or the leader of the Slavic-Orthodox civilization has been a recurring one in Russian history. That issue was obscured by the communist victory in Russia, which imported a Western ideology, adapted it to Russian conditions and then challenged the West in the name of that ideology. The dominance of communism shut off the historic debate over Westernization versus Russification. With communism discredited Russians once again face that question.

President Yeltsin is adopting Western principles and goals and seeking to make Russia a "normal" country and a part of the West. Yet both the Russian elite and the Russian public are divided on this issue. Among the more moderate dissenters, Sergei Stankevich argues that Russia should reject the "Atlanticist" course, which would lead it "to become European, to become a part of the world economy in rapid and organized fashion, to become the eighth member of the Seven, and to particular emphasis on Germany and the United States as the two dominant members of the Atlantic alliance." While also rejecting an exclusively Eurasian policy, Stankevich nonetheless argues that Russia should give priority to the protection of Russians in other countries, emphasize its Turkic and Muslim connections, and promote "an appreciable redistribution of our resources, our options, our ties, and our interests in favor of Asia, of the eastern direction." People of this persuasion criticize Yeltsin for subordinating Russia's interests to those of the West, for reducing Russian military strength, for failing to support traditional friends such as Serbia, and for pushing economic and political reform in ways injurious to the Russian people. Indicative of this trend is the new popularity of the ideas of Petr Savitsky, who in the 1920s argued that Russia was a unique Eurasian civilization. (7) More extreme dissidents voice much more blatantly nationalist, anti-Western and anti-Semitic views, and urge Russia to redevelop its military strength and to establish closer ties with China and Muslim countries. The people of Russia areas divided as the elite. An opinion survey in European Russia in the spring of 1992 revealed that 40 percent of the public had positive attitudes toward the West and 36 percent had negative attitudes. As it has been for much of its history, Russia in the early 1990s is truly a torn country.

To redefine its civilization identity, a torn country must meet three requirements. First, its political and economic elite has to be generally supportive of and enthusiastic about the move. Second, its public has to be willing to acquiesce in the redefinition. Third, the dominant groups in the recipient civilization have to be willing to embrace the convert. All three requirements in large part exist with respect to Mexico. The first two in large part exist with respect to Turkey. It is not clear that any of them exist with respect to Russia's joining the West. The conflict between liberal democracy and Marxism-Leninism was between ideologies which, despite their major differences, ostensibly shared ultimate goals of freedom, equality and prosperity. A traditional, authoritarian, nationalist Russia could have quite different goals. A Western democrat could carry on an intellectual debate with a Soviet Marxist. It would be virtually impossible for him to do that with a Russian traditionalist. If, as the Russians stop behaving like Marxists, they reject liberal democracy and begin behaving like Russians but not like Westerners, the relations between Russia and the West could again become distant and conflictual. (8)

Australia's future, they argue, is with the dynamic economies of East Asia. But, as I have suggested, close economic cooperation normally requires a common cultural base. In addition, none of the three conditions necessary for a torn country to join another civilization is likely to exist in Australia's case.

VIII. The Confucian-Islamic Connection

The obstacles to non-Western countries joining the West vary considerably. They are least for Latin American and East European countries. They are greater for the Orthodox countries of the former Soviet Union. They are still greater for Muslim, Confucian, Hindu and Buddhist societies. Japan has established a unique position for itself as an associate member of the West: it is in the West in some respects but clearly not of the West in important dimensions. Those countries that for reason of culture and power do not wish to, or cannot, join the West compete with the West by developing their own economic, military and political power. They do this by promoting their internal development and by cooperating with other non-Western countries. The most prominent form of this cooperation is the Confucian-Islamic connection that has emerged to challenge Western interests, values and power.

Almost without exception, Western countries are reducing their military power; under Yeltsin's leadership so also is Russia. China, North Korea and several Middle Eastern states, however, are significantly expanding their military capabilities. They are doing this by the import of arms from Western and non-Western sources and by the development of indigenous arms industries. One result is the emergence of what Charles Krauthammer has called "Weapon States," and the Weapon States are not Western states. Another result is the redefinition of arms control, which is a Western concept and a Western goal. During the Cold War the primary purpose of arms control was to establish a stable military balance between the United States and its allies and the Soviet Union and its allies. In the post-Cold War world the primary objective of arms control is to prevent the development by non-Western societies of military capabilities that could threaten Western interests. The West attempts to do this through international agreements, economic pressure and controls on the transfer of arms and weapons technologies.

The conflict between the West and the Confucian-Islamic states focuses largely, although not exclusively, on nuclear, chemical and biological weapons, ballistic missiles and other sophisticated means for delivering them, and the guidance, intelligence and other electronic capabilities for achieving that goal. The West promotes nonproliferation as a universal norm and nonproliferation treaties and inspections as means of realizing that norm. It also threatens a variety of sanctions against those who promote the spread of sophisticated weapons and proposes some benefits for those who do not. The attention of the West focuses, naturally on nations that are actually or potentially hostile to the West.

The non-Western nations, on the other hand, assert their right to acquire and to deploy whatever weapons they think necessary for their security. They also have absorbed, to the full, the truth of the response of the Indian defense minister when asked what lesson he learned from the Gulf War: "Don't fight the United States unless you have nuclear weapons." Nuclear weapons, chemical weapons and missiles are viewed, probably erroneously, as the potential equalizer of superior Western conventional power. China, of course, already has nuclear weapons; Pakistan and India have the capability to deploy them. North Korea, Iran, Iraq, Libya and Algeria appear to be attempting to acquire them. A top Iranian official has declared that all Muslim states should acquire nuclear weapons, and in 1988 the president of Iran reportedly issued a directive calling for development of "offensive and defensive chemical, biological and radiological weapons."

Centrally important to the development of counter-West military capabilities is the sustained expansion of China's military power and its means to create military power. Buoyed by spectacular economic development, China is rapidly increasing its military spending and vigorously moving forward with the modernization of its armed forces. It is purchasing weapons from the former Soviet states; it is developing long-range missiles; in 1992 it tested a one-megaton nuclear device. It is developing power-projection capabilities, acquiring aerial refueling technology, and trying to purchase an aircraft carrier. Its military buildup and assertion of sovereignty over the South China Sea are provoking a multilateral regional arms race in East Asia. China is also a major exporter of arms and weapons technology.

It has exported materials to Libya and Iraq that could be used to manufacture nuclear weapons and nerve gas. It has helped Algeria build a reactor suitable for nuclear weapons research and production. China has sold to Iran nuclear technology that American officials believe could only be used to create weapons and apparently has shipped components of 300-mile-range missiles to Pakistan. North Korea has had a nuclear weapons program under way for some while and has sold advanced missiles and missile technology to Syria and Iran. The flow of weapons and weapons technology is generally from East Asia to the Middle East.

There is, however, some movement in the reverse direction; China has received Stinger missiles from Pakistan. A Confucian-Islamic military connection has thus come into being, designed to promote acquisition by its members of the weapons and weapons technologies needed to counter the military powers of the West. It may or may not last. At present, however, it is, as Dave McCurdy has said, "a renegades' mutual support pact, run by the proliferators and their backers." A new form of arms competition is thus occurring between Islamic-Confucian states and the West. In an old-fashioned arms race, each side developed its own arms to balance or to achieve superiority against the other side. In this new form of arms competition, one side is developing its arms and the other side is attempting not to balance but to limit and prevent that arms build-up while at the same time reducing its own military capabilities.

IX. Implications for the West

This ar ticle does not argue that civilization identities will replace all other identities, that nation states will disappear, that each civilization will become a single coherent political entity, that groups within a civilization will not conflict with and even fight each other. This paper does set forth the hypotheses that differences between civilizations are real and important; civilization-consciousness is increasing; conflict between civilizations will supplant ideological and other forms of conflict as the dominant global form of conflict; international relations, historically a game played out within Western civilization, will increasingly be de-Westernized and become a game in which non-Western civilizations are actors and not simply objects; successful political, security and economic international institutions are more likely to develop within civilizations than across civilizations; conflicts between groups in different civilizations will be more frequent, more sustained and more violent than conflicts between groups in the same civilization; violent conflicts between groups in different civilizations are the most likely and most dangerous source of escalation that could lead to global wars; the paramount axis of world politics will be the relations between "the West and the Rest"; the elites in some torn non-Western countries will try to make their countries part of the West, but in most cases face major obstacles to accomplishing this; a central focus of conflict for the immediate future will be between the West and several Islamic-Confucian states.

This is not to advocate the desirability of conflicts between civilizations. It is to set forth descriptive hypotheses as to what the future may be like. If these are plausible hypotheses, however, it is necessary to consider their implications for Western policy. These implications should be divided between short-term advantage and long-term accommodation. In the short term it is clearly in the interest of the West to promote greater cooperation and unity within its own civilization, particularly between its European and North American components; to incorporate into the West societies in Eastern Europe and Latin America whose cultures are close to those of the West; to promote and maintain cooperative relations with Russia and Japan; to prevent escalation of local inter-civilization conflicts into major inter-civilization wars; to limit the expansion of the military strength of Confucian and Islamic states; to moderate the reduction of counter military capabilities and maintain military superiority in East and Southwest Asia; to exploit differences and conflicts among Confucian and Islamic states; to support in other civilizations groups sympathetic to Western values and interests; to strengthen international institutions that reflect and legitimate Western interests and values and to promote the involvement of non-Western states in those institutions.

In the longer term other measures would be called for. Western civilization is both Western and modern. Non-Western civilizations have attempted to become modern without becoming Western. To date only Japan has fully succeeded in this quest. Non-Western civilization will continue to attempt to acquire the wealth, technology, skills, machines and weapons that are part of being modern. They will also attempt to reconcile this modernity with their traditional culture and values. Their economic and military strength relative to the West will increase. Hence the West will increasingly have to accommodate these non-Western modern civilizations whose power approaches that of the West but whose values and interests differ significantly from those of the West. This will require the West to maintain the economic and military power necessary to protect its interests in relation to these civilizations. It will also, however, require the West to develop a more profound understanding of the basic religious and philosophical assumptions underlying other civilizations and the ways in which people in those civilizations see their interests. It will require an effort to identify elements of commonality between Western and other civilizations. For the relevant future, there will be no universal civilization, but instead a world of different civilizations, each of which will have to learn to coexist with the others.

(1) Murray Weidenbaum, Greater China: The Next Economic Superpower?, St. Louis: Washington University Center for the Study of American Business, Contemporary Issues, Series 57, February 1993, pp. 2-3.

(2) Bernard Lewis, "The Roots of Muslim Rage," The Atlantic Monthly, vol. 266, September 1990, p. 60; Time, June 15, 1992, pp. 24-28.

(3) Archie Roosevelt, For Lust of Knowing, Boston: Little, Brown, 1988, PP 332-333.

(4) Almost invariably Western leaders claim they are acting on behalf of "the world community." One minor lapse occurred during the run-up to the Gulf War. In an interview on "Good Morning America," Dec. 21, 1990, British Prime Minister John Major referred to the actions "the West" was taking against Saddam Hussein. He quickly corrected himself and subsequently referred to "the world community." He was, however, right when he erred.

(5) Harry C. Triandis, The New York Times, Dec. 25, 1990, p. 41, and "Cross-Cultural Studies of Individualism and Collectivism," Nebraska Symposium on Motivation, vol. 37, 1989, pp. 41-133.

(6) Kishore Mahbubani, "The West and the Rest," The National Interest, Summer 1992, pp. 3-13.

(7) Sergei Stankevich, "Russia in Search of Itself," The National Interest, Summer 1992, pp. 47-51; Daniel Schneider, "A Russian Movement Rejects Western Tilt," Christian Science Monitor, Feb. 5, 1993, pp. 5-7.

(8) Owen Harries has pointed out that Australia is trying (unwisely in his view) to become a torn country in reverse. Although it has been a full member

not only of the West but also of the ABCA military and intelligence core of the West, its current leaders are in effect proposing that it defect from the West, redefine itself as an Asian country and cultivate dose ties with its neighbors. Australia's future, they argue, is with the dynamic economies of East Asia. But, as I have suggested, close economic cooperation normally requires a common cultural base. In addition, none of the three conditions necessary for a torn country to join another civilization is likely to exist in Australia's case.

Writing Alone

1. b "Muslims Staking out Their Place in Europe"

by Evan Osnos, Chicago Tribune

There has been much talked and written about in recent years about changing worldwide demographics; we see it in the United States with the rise of Hispanic populations.

- Do you think what Osnos proposes about Muslim immigration to Europe is a real or imagined threat?

- Is the author an alarmist? Just reporting the news?

- Can you relate to any of the scenes Osnos creates?

- Will changing demographics in the United States alter the political landscape? Affect social stability?

ST.-DENIS, France - (KRT) - Butchered piglets hang in tidy rows at the open-air market, and shoppers haggle over cheese and oysters in a scene hardly altered since the last Bourbon king was buried at the Gothic church on the corner. But slip out of the market on a Friday, and a quarter-mile up the road you will find a very different France: Hundreds of Muslims squeezed hip to hip into an unheated canvas tent, bowing in sacred silence toward Mecca, the birthplace of Islam, which few of them have ever seen.

The worshipers at this makeshift mosque on the edge of Paris are men and women, dressed in the latest fashions and traditional robes, Arab, European and African. They are moderate, conservative and fundamentalist. They are first-, second- and third-generation immigrants. They are content and they are enraged. They are the future that Europe is straining to handle.

What is happening in Europe may provide a partial preview of what lies ahead for the United States and its fast-growing Muslim population.

For the first time in history, Muslims are building large and growing minorities across the secular Western world - nowhere more visibly than in Western Europe, where their numbers have more than doubled in the past two decades. The impact is unfolding from Amsterdam to Paris to Madrid, as Muslims struggle - with words, votes and sometimes violence - to stake out their place in adopted societies. Disproportionately young, poor and unemployed, they seek greater recognition and an Islam that fits their lives. Just as Egypt, Pakistan and Iran are witnessing the debate over the shape of Islam today, Europe is emerging as the battleground of tomorrow.

"The French are scared," said Tair Abdelkader, 38, a regular at the tented mosque whose light blue eyes and ebony beard are the legacy of a French mother and Algerian father. "In 10 years, the Muslim community will be stronger and stronger, and French political culture must accept that."

By midcentury, at least one in five Europeans will be Muslim. That change is unlike other waves of immigration because it poses a more essential challenge: defining a modern Judeo-Christian-Islamic civilization. The West must decide how its laws and values will shape and be shaped by Islam.

For Europe, as well as the United States, the question is not which civilization, Western or Islamic, will prevail, but which of Islam's many strands will dominate. Will it be compatible with Western values or will it reject them?

Center stage in that debate is France, home to the largest Islamic community on the continent, an estimated 5 million Muslims. Here the process of defining Euro-Islam is unfolding around questions as concrete as the right to wear head scarves and as abstract as the meaning of citizenship, secularism and extremism. In some cases, conservative Muslims have refused to visit co-ed swimming pools, study Darwinism or allow women to be examined by male doctors.

One young St.-Denis fundamentalist recently set off for Iraq and was captured fighting American troops in Fallujah. Stunned by stories like that, France is hoping to use the legal system to influence the direction of Islam within its borders. The government has deported 84 people in the past six months on suspicion of advocating violence and drawn wide attention for banning head scarves and other religious symbols in public school. But even supporters of that tough approach concede that the measures can do little more than patch the widening cracks in Europe's image of itself.

"I'm not sure we'll go much further than gaining a few months or years" in the effort to limit Islam's imprint on France, said Herve Mariton, a member of the French Parliament who lobbied for the head scarf law. "That may be useful. But there is no way this is the ultimate answer to the challenge."

St.-Denis' narrow streets sweep outward from a soaring 12th century basilica that is the final resting place for generations of French monarchs. But today their snowy stone statues stare down onto a city and nation in transformation.

The Muslim migration to Europe began in earnest after World War II, when North African workers arrived by the thousands to help rebuild the continent. A half-century later, no fewer than a third of St.-Denis' 90,000 residents are of Arab origin. Arabic script on butcher shops and storefronts touts halal meat, handled to Islamic standards. Couscous restaurants are as plentiful as brasseries. Muslim settlement houses usher in new immigrants, and Muslim funeral homes bid farewell to old ones.

Across the country, French Muslims still live more or less where the first arrivals settled a half-century ago, in suburban apartment blocks erected in the 1950s for foreign workers. These suburbs, the banlieues, have become the byword for France's virtually segregated Muslim communities. The complexes used to be integrated, with Polish, Italian and French workers living among North African arrivals, but over time the Europeans moved on - and the Arabs did not. It is a scene repeated across the suburbs of Paris.

"Gradually the French people left or died, and they were replaced by more people from North Africa," said Brigitte Fouvez, 55, deputy mayor in the neighboring town of Bondy. "The French people who stayed would say, `You can smell the cooking in the hallways,' and eventually they left too."

Like other ethnic Europeans, Fouvez and her husband moved from Paris in 1978 in search of more room for their two children. She watched Bondy evolve. "Before, we had a charcuterie and a butcher," she said. "Now there are just three halal butchers, no fish shop anymore, no traditional French stores." But those changes weren't nearly as startling as the sight of conservative Muslim women draped head to toe in dark chador robes - to Fouvez's eyes, "as black as crows."

Thirteen hundred years after the Frankish King Charles Martel repelled Muslim armies from the central city of Tours, Islam is now the second religion of France; there are about 10 times as many Muslims as Jews.

From the Paris suburbs 25 years ago, Shiite Ayatollah Ruhollah Khomeini planned a revolution that ultimately overthrew the Shah of Iran and, in turn, helped inspire a global Islamic revival. The fallout is easily visible today as the children and grandchildren of Muslim immigrants in Europe increasingly embrace religion. In France and England, polls show greater commitment to daily prayers, mosque attendance and fasting during Ramadan than there was a decade ago.

Only one in five Muslims in France say they actively practice the faith, but many who once defined themselves in terms of Tunisian, Iraqi or Turkish descent now consider their primary identity to be Muslim. "Nobody was talking about Muslims in France at the end of the 1990s. People were talking about Arabs or beurs," said French political scientist Justin Vaisse, using the term applied to French of North African immigrant descent.

Young French Muslims gravitate toward charismatic spokesmen of a new European Islam, such as controversial Swiss-born philosopher Tariq Ramadan, whose French headquarters here in St.-Denis urges a "silent revolution." In his writings, he advocates using the political process, instead of violence, to win

Muslim rights and recognition across Europe. Ramadan's supporters call him a major voice of moderate Islam, but some critics say he is tied to extremists, a charge he denies. He was scheduled to begin teaching this year at the University of Notre Dame until U.S. immigration authorities rescinded his work visa, citing unspecified national security concerns.

Unlike earlier immigrants, who were bent on returning home flush with cash, more-recent arrivals have been deterred by the turmoil in their homelands and stayed, building families that are larger than those of their graying ethnic European neighbors. The effect is amplified by the decline of European Christianity. The number of people who call themselves Catholic, the continent's largest denomination, has declined by more than a third in the past 25 years. The results are stark. Within six years, for instance, the three largest cities in the Netherlands will be majority Muslim. One-third of all German Muslims are younger than 18, nearly twice the proportion of the general population.

With that growth, and the deepening strains between the U.S. and the Islamic world, radical Muslim clerics have found no shortage of adherents. A 2002 poll of British Muslims found that 44 percent believe attacks by al-Qaida are justified as long as "Muslims are being killed by America and its allies using American weapons." Germany estimates that there are 31,000 Islamists in the country, based on membership lists of conservative federations.

Year by year, European Islam pulls further away from the cultural traditions of Morocco or Algeria, refashioned all the while by the pressures of life in Europe. For some, the solution is a more liberalized Islam that incorporates Western concepts of individual rights and tolerance. But for others, the answer lies in a stricter interpretation of the core elements of the faith. "It is more fundamentalist in its essence because what you subsist on is personal practice_reading of the Koran, Shariah," Vaisse said. "It can take very humanist forms, but in some cases, it can also lead to political radicalization and terrorism."

The potentially serious effects of that radicalization became clear on March 11, when coordinated bombings of four commuter trains in Madrid killed 191 people and wounded more than 1,800. Moroccan and Tunisian suspects later killed themselves in a standoff with police. More recently, the Netherlands is in turmoil after the brutal killing of Theo van Gogh, who made a controversial film about violence against women in Islamic societies. Police arrested a 26-year-old man with Dutch-Moroccan citizenship and charged him with stabbing and shooting van Gogh. The suspect allegedly pinned a note to the body with a knife.

Within days, an Islamic school was set ablaze, and retribution followed. Right-wing politicians in Belgium and Germany demanded new curbs on immigration. In time, however, a more ominous fact emerged from the case: It was not the work of newly arrived immigrants with extremist views, but the product of homegrown radicalism. Police say suspect Mohammed Bouyeri wrote the death note in Dutch, not Arabic.

"This (cultural) schizophrenia is the most dangerous thing we face in Europe today," said Gilles Kepel, head of Middle East studies at the Institute of Political Studies in Paris and author of several books on Islam in Europe. "It means Madrid. It means Mohamed Atta," he said, referring to one of the Sept. 11 hijackers who lived for some time in Germany.

Where moderate Muslims ultimately place their loyalty may be the defining - and unpredictable - ingredient in the struggle to fashion an Islam of the West. To understand the choices, visit the men who represent the two competing visions of Islam in France. Dalil Boubakeur, rector of the Grand Mosque of Paris in the heart of the city, is a long-standing voice of moderate Islam in France. On the other side is Lhaj Thami Breze, president of the Union of Islamic Organizations of France, the increasingly powerful Islamist federation.

Trained as a dentist, Boubakeur, 64, runs the 1920s-era mosque in the heart Paris. He is prone to quoting Immanuel Kant and is a favorite of French officials and foreign ambassadors. He wears a red rosebud on his lapel signifying membership in the Legion of Honor. And he knows he is losing ground. "Since Sept. 11, the world of Islam is changing faster in the West than other places in the world," he said at his antiques-lined office, his V-neck sweater, rimless glasses and wispy gray hair giving him the air of an English schoolmaster. "Western countries had had a gentleman's agreement with fundamentalists: You can stay here as long as you keep quiet. But the gentlemen are not being as quiet as they used to be."

There is no question that Boubakeur's influence is weakening. Last year he was handpicked to be president of the official French Council of the Muslim Faith, a new body established by the government in 2003 to give Muslims a formal voice in dealings with the state. Just as other bodies represent Catholics and Jews, the council speaks for Muslims on issues such as the construction of mosques and the training of clerics. But things didn't go as planned. In the first election, his moderate camp was trounced by conservative candidates who won 70 percent of the 41 seats. The next vote is scheduled for April, and moderates are expected to lose even more to the men he believes are "radicalizing Islam" in France.

"The facts are there: Religions that close in on themselves become sects, and that is what is happening to Islam here," Boubakeur said. "And I am very sorry about that."

Across town, beside the highway in the tough Paris suburb of La Courneuve, Boubakeur's opponents are confident. Breze greets visitors at his glass-and-steel headquarters with a glossy package of materials and a calm message of "coordination, not confrontation."

"We are not extremists," he says, sipping espresso at a conference table. "We practice our beliefs and have respect for the state. We want one thing from Europe and France: that they are faithful to their values."

Indeed, Breze and the union have thrived under Western democracy. Just two decades after its creation, by two foreign students, the union dominates French Islam. In the last elections for the Council of the Muslim Faith, Breze won control of a crucial post representing central France. Breze's federation draws 30,000 people to its annual conference, and the crowd is increasingly vocal in challenging the political powers that be. At last year's convention, the interior minister was booed in the middle of his speech when he suggested that women must remove their head scarves for ID photos.

So what does Breze really want for Muslims in France? He and his group carefully calibrate their demands. They demonstrate against the ban on head scarves, for instance, but urge young women to respect the law as long as it is in effect. His federation is part of a broader umbrella group for all of Europe that is known for issuing decisions that help conservative Muslims function in a modern Western society by permitting, for instance, interest-bearing loans that would otherwise be banned under Islam and allowing the consumption of pork-based gelatin.

Push Breze on the most sensitive issues - does he seek an Islamic state in France, or the application of strict Islamic law and punishment - and he says no: "Perhaps they are valid in Saudi Arabia or Palestine, but they are not valid here." To some critics, Breze is a "double talker" who says one thing in French and another in Arabic. To others, he is simply a shrewd strategist who understands the coming power of the fast-growing Muslim communities here. For his part, Breze says his mission is to convey a simple message: "France must respect this population."

By all appearances, she is as French as they come. A law student at the Sorbonne, she has dark brown hair that falls in stylish curls to her shoulders. Dining with friends in downtown Paris, 23-year-old Faten Mansour wears Diesel-brand jeans and red stiletto heels. But she will be the first to point out that she is not just French.

"I am a woman, I am an Arab and I come from the suburbs. I have three handicaps," she says. "France is not racist, but it is xenophobic. I can study the law all night, but I don't know if I will find a job - not because I'm not competent, but because I'm an Arab."

That feeling of exclusion has emerged as the central issue in the struggle to integrate Islam in Europe. Whether it is Turks in Germany, Indonesians in the Netherlands or Pakistanis in Britain, polls show Muslims feel they live in a parallel world within Europe. There are no Muslims in the French Parliament, no Muslim CEOs of top French companies, and the national news media is overwhelmingly white. Midlevel Muslim politicians routinely recite instances of their careers being diverted by higher-ups.

In an unusually blunt official assessment, the French government's auditing agency in a report released Nov. 23 faulted the republic for failing to combat segregation in housing, workplaces and schools. The same week, France's largest insurer, AXA, presented a report concluding that young immigrants in France experience a rate of unemployment that is 2 to 5 times as high as that of young people who are ethnic European.

Moreover, that frustration is getting worse over time. "The first generation came to Europe to work, the second generation was caught in between two cultures. But the third generation is completely French, and they want all the rights of citizenship," said Khalid Bouchama, the St.-Denis representative for Breze's group. For ethnic Europeans, the Muslim migration amounts to a world upended: The continent that for centuries exported its people, culture and religion to the Third World is now being shaped by its former colonies. But for the French establishment, the challenge is to bring Muslims into European society without changing the foundations of secular democracy.

No decision has sparked more controversy than the French government's move to ban conspicuous religious symbols from public schools, including Muslim head scarves, Jewish yarmulkes and large crosses. To its opponents, the law was a blunt refusal to accept Muslim immigration. But to its supporters, it was a decisive move to lower the barriers building between France's young people.

"It showed you can only go so far, you can't go any further," said Blandine Kriegel, an adviser to President Jacques Chirac on integration issues. "The issue touched a raw nerve. It is a nerve that is at the very heart of our way of life."

Kepel, the professor, served on the commission that recommended the law. He originally opposed the idea, he says, until he heard testimony from teachers and young women who described how young fundamentalists used girls' decisions to wear a veil as leverage to pressure them into adopting a more religious lifestyle.

"If we were accused of being Islamaphobes, let's take it and not give a damn. It was a time to give those kids the opportunities to interact in the best possible way and not jeopardize their futures in French society," Kepel said.

French Muslims responded with mass protests. Terrorists in Iraq abducted two French journalists and demanded that the law be repealed or the captives would be killed. The move backfired - French Muslims roundly denounced the threat. The journalists were returned this week. Four months into the first school year under the law, 45 girls across France remain out of school or in mediation over their refusal to remove their scarves. Considering that 2,000 girls were believed to be wearing the veil last year, French officials have been pleased with the outcome.

Other than the veil law, Kriegel said, the government is trying to reduce segregation of Muslim immigrants by expanding access to French language instruction and combating workplace discrimination. The government, she believes, is on the right track. "There are no fires in the banlieues," she said. "There are no riots as there were in the black ghettos in the United States in the 1960s. Why don't we have that? Because we've been rolling up our sleeves and doing something. ... We have turned the corner."

But in St.-Denis and other suburbs, the verdict is less clear. The huddles of young men stand like emblems of 17 percent unemployment, well above the national average. Classrooms and public housing are overcrowded with fast-growing immigrant families. The mosques are busier than ever: the storefront Tawhid Center for young followers of Tariq Ramadan; the Tabligh mosque for the reclusive adherents of Saudi-style conservative Islam; the many basement prayer rooms for whoever stops by.

A French intelligence official who monitors fundamentalist groups said he believes the veil controversy and efforts to train imams have pushed French Muslims to an awkward reckoning point: They must decide whether to integrate with Europe or fight back in earnest against official efforts to shape their community. "They are at a crossroads," he said. "They can either go left or right."

Evaluating Sources

1.c. "The Coming Wars: What the Pentagon Can Now do in Secret"

by Seymour M. Hersh

> *Seymour Myron (Sy) Hersh (1937) is an American Pulitzer Prize winning investigative journalist and author based in New York City. He is a regular contributor to The New Yorker on military and security matters. His work first gained worldwide recognition in 1969 for exposing the My Lai massacre and its cover-up during the Vietnam War, for which he received the 1970 Pulitzer Prize for International Reporting. His 2004 reports on the US Military's treatment of detainees at Abu Ghraib prison gained much attention. In 2006, he reported on the US military's plans for Iran, which called for the use of nuclear weapons against that country.*

While reading the next essay, try to evaluate Hersh's sources:

- Who are the sources of Hersh's information?

- Are they credible? Does it sound like hearsay?

- Can you determine if the author is biased in his politics? If the author is unbiased and reporting the facts, what is the author's Outlook? Forecast?

- Do you agree with the author? Are you alarmed by the message, or is it just another voice for you?

George W. Bush's reëlection was not his only victory last fall. The President and his national-security advisers have consolidated control over the military and intelligence communities' strategic analyses and covert operations to a degree unmatched since the rise of the post-Second World War national-security state. Bush has an aggressive and ambitious agenda for using that control—against the mullahs in Iran and against targets in the ongoing war on terrorism—during his second term. The C.I.A. will continue to be downgraded, and the agency will increasingly serve, as one government consultant with close ties to the Pentagon put it, as "facilitators" of policy emanating from President Bush and Vice-President Dick Cheney. This process is well under way.

Despite the deteriorating security situation in Iraq, the Bush Administration has not reconsidered its basic long-range policy goal in the Middle East: the establishment of democracy throughout the region. Bush's reëlection is regarded within the Administration as evidence of America's support for his decision to go to war. It has reaffirmed the position of the neoconservatives in the Pentagon's civilian leadership who advocated the invasion, including Paul Wolfowitz, the Deputy Secretary of Defense, and Douglas Feith, the Under-secretary for Policy. According to a former high-level intelligence official, Secretary of Defense Donald Rumsfeld met with the Joint Chiefs of Staff shortly after the election and told them, in essence, that the naysayers had been heard and the American people did not accept their message. Rumsfeld added that America was committed to staying in Iraq and that there would be no second-guessing.

"This is a war against terrorism, and Iraq is just one campaign. The Bush Administration is looking at this as a huge war zone," the former high-level intelligence official told me. "Next, we're going to have the Iranian campaign. We've declared war and the bad guys, wherever they are, are the enemy. This is the last hurrah—we've got four years, and want to come out of this saying we won the war on terrorism."

Bush and Cheney may have set the policy, but it is Rumsfeld who has directed its implementation and has absorbed much of the public criticism when things went wrong—whether it was prisoner abuse in Abu Ghraib or lack of sufficient armor plating for G.I.s' vehicles in Iraq. Both Democratic and Republican lawmakers have called for Rumsfeld's dismissal, and he is not widely admired inside the military. Nonetheless, his reappointment as Defense Secretary was never in doubt.

Rumsfeld will become even more important during the second term. In interviews with past and present intelligence and military officials, I was told that the agenda had been determined before the Presidential election, and much of it would be Rumsfeld's responsibility. The war on terrorism would be expanded, and effectively placed under the Pentagon's control. The President has signed a series of findings and executive orders authorizing secret commando groups and other Special Forces units to conduct covert operations against suspected terrorist targets in as many as ten nations in the Middle East and South Asia.

The President's decision enables Rumsfeld to run the operations off the books—free from legal restrictions imposed on the C.I.A. Under current law, all C.I.A. covert activities overseas must be authorized by a Presidential finding and reported to the Senate and House intelligence committees. (The laws were enacted after a series of scandals in the nineteen-seventies involving C.I.A. domestic spying and attempted assassinations of foreign leaders.) "The Pentagon doesn't feel obligated to report any of this to Congress," the former high-level intelligence official said. "They don't even call it 'covert ops'—it's too close to the C.I.A. phrase. In their view, it's 'black reconnaissance.' They're not even going to tell the cincs"— the regional American military commanders-in-chief. (The Defense Department and the White House did not respond to requests for comment on this story.)

In my interviews, I was repeatedly told that the next strategic target was Iran. "Everyone is saying, 'You can't be serious about targeting Iran. Look at Iraq,'" the former intelligence official told me. "But they say, 'We've got some lessons learned—not militarily, but how we did it politically. We're not going to rely on agency pissants.' No loose ends, and that's why the C.I.A. is out of there."

For more than a year, France, Germany, Britain, and other countries in the European Union have seen preventing Iran from getting a nuclear weapon as a race against time—and against the Bush Administration. They have been negotiating with the Iranian leadership to give up its nuclear-weapons ambitions in exchange for economic aid and trade benefits. Iran has agreed to temporarily halt its enrichment programs, which generate fuel for nuclear power plants but also could produce weapons-grade fissile material. (Iran claims that such facilities are legal under the Nuclear Non-Proliferation Treaty, or N.P.T., to which it is a signator, and that it has no intention of building a bomb.) But the goal of the current round of talks, which began in December in Brussels, is to persuade Tehran to go further, and dismantle its machinery. Iran insists, in return, that it needs to see some concrete benefits from the Europeans—oil-production technology, heavy-industrial equipment, and perhaps even permission to purchase a fleet of Airbuses. (Iran has been denied access to technology and many goods owing to sanctions.)

The Europeans have been urging the Bush Administration to join in these negotiations. The Administration has refused to do so. The civilian leadership in the Pentagon has argued that no diplomatic progress on the Iranian nuclear threat will take place unless there is a credible threat of military action. "The neocons say negotiations are a bad deal," a senior official of the International Atomic Energy Agency (I.A.E.A.) told me. "And the only thing the Iranians understand is pressure. And that they also need to be whacked."

The core problem is that Iran has successfully hidden the extent of its nuclear program, and its progress. Many Western intelligence agencies, including those of the United States, believe that Iran is at least three to five years away from a capability to independently produce nuclear warheads—although its work on a missile-delivery system is far more advanced. Iran is also widely believed by Western intelligence agencies and the I.A.E.A. to have serious technical problems with its weapons system, most notably in the production of the hexafluoride gas needed to fabricate nuclear warheads.

A retired senior C.I.A. official, one of many who left the agency recently, told me that he was familiar with the assessments, and confirmed that Iran is known to be having major difficulties in its weapons work. He also acknowledged that the agency's timetable for a nuclear Iran matches the European estimates—assuming that Iran gets no outside help. "The big wild card for us is that you don't know who is capable of filling in the missing parts for them," the recently retired official said. "North Korea? Pakistan? We don't know what parts are missing."

One Western diplomat told me that the Europeans believed they were in what he called a "lose-lose position" as long as the United States refuses to get involved. "France, Germany, and the U.K. cannot succeed alone, and everybody knows it," the diplomat said. "If the U.S. stays outside, we don't have enough leverage, and our effort will collapse." The alternative would be to go to the Security Council, but any resolution imposing sanctions would likely be vetoed by China or Russia, and then "the United Nations will be blamed and the Americans will say, 'The only solution is to bomb.'"

A European Ambassador noted that President Bush is scheduled to visit Europe in February, and that there has been public talk from the White House about improving the President's relationship with America's E.U. allies. In that context, the Ambassador told me, "I'm puzzled by the fact that the United States is not helping us in our program. How can Washington maintain its stance without seriously taking into account the weapons issue?"

The Israeli government is, not surprisingly, skeptical of the European approach. Silvan Shalom, the Foreign Minister, said in an interview last week in Jerusalem,with another New Yorker journalist, "I don't like what's happening. We were encouraged at first when the Europeans got involved. For a long time, they thought it was just Israel's problem. But then they saw that the [Iranian] missiles themselves were longer range and could reach all of Europe, and they became very concerned. Their attitude has been to use the carrot and the stick—but all we see so far is the carrot." He added, "If they can't comply, Israel cannot live with Iran having a nuclear bomb."

In a recent essay, Patrick Clawson, an Iran expert who is the deputy director of the Washington Institute for Near East Policy (and a supporter of the Administration), articulated the view that force, or the threat of it, was a vital bargaining tool with Iran. Clawson wrote that if Europe wanted coöperation with the Bush Administration it "would do well to remind Iran that the military option remains on the table." He added that the argument that the European negotiations hinged on Washington looked like "a preëmptive excuse for the likely breakdown of the E.U.-Iranian talks." In a subsequent conversation with me, Clawson suggested that, if some kind of military action was inevitable, "it would be much more in Israel's interest—and Washington's—to take covert action. The style of this Administration is to use overwhelming force—'shock and awe.' But we get only one bite of the apple."

There are many military and diplomatic experts who dispute the notion that military action, on whatever scale, is the right approach. Shahram Chubin, an Iranian scholar who is the director of research at the Geneva Centre for Security Policy, told me, "It's a fantasy to think that there's a good American or Israeli military option in Iran." He went on, "The Israeli view is that this is an international problem. 'You do it,' they say to the West. 'Otherwise, our Air Force will take care of it.'" In 1981, the Israeli Air Force destroyed Iraq's Osirak reactor, setting its nuclear program back several years. But the situation now is both more complex and more dangerous, Chubin said. The Osirak bombing "drove the Iranian nuclear-weapons program underground, to hardened, dispersed sites," he said. "You can't be sure after an attack that you'll get away with it. The U.S. and Israel would not be certain whether all the sites had been hit, or how quickly they'd be rebuilt. Meanwhile, they'd be waiting for an Iranian counter-attack that could be military or terrorist or diplomatic. Iran has long-range missiles and ties to Hezbollah, which has drones—you can't begin to think of what they'd do in response."

Chubin added that Iran could also renounce the Nuclear Non-Proliferation Treaty. "It's better to have them cheating within the system," he said. "Otherwise, as victims, Iran will walk away from the treaty and inspections while the rest of the world watches the N.P.T. unravel before their eyes."

The Administration has been conducting secret reconnaissance missions inside Iran at least since last summer. Much of the focus is on the accumulation of intelligence and targeting information on Iranian nuclear, chemical, and missile sites, both declared and suspected. The goal is to identify and isolate three dozen, and perhaps more, such targets that could be destroyed by precision strikes and short-term commando raids. "The civilians in the Pentagon want to go into Iran and destroy as much of the military infrastructure as possible," the government consultant with close ties to the Pentagon told me.

Some of the missions involve extraordinary coöperation. For example, the former high-level intelligence official told me that an American commando task force has been set up in South Asia and is now working closely with a group of Pakistani scientists and technicians who had dealt with Iranian counterparts. (In 2003, the I.A.E.A. disclosed that Iran had been secretly receiving nuclear technology from Pakistan for more than a decade, and had withheld that information from inspectors.) The American task force, aided by the information from Pakistan, has been penetrating eastern Iran from Afghanistan in a hunt for underground installations. The task-force members, or their locally recruited agents, secreted remote detection devices—known as sniffers—capable of sampling the atmosphere for radioactive emissions and other evidence of nuclear-enrichment programs.

Getting such evidence is a pressing concern for the Bush Administration. The former high-level intelligence official told me, "They don't want to make any W.M.D. intelligence mistakes, as in Iraq. The Republicans can't have two of those. There's no education in the second kick of a mule." The official added that the government of Pervez Musharraf, the Pakistani President, has won a high price for its coöperation—American assurance that Pakistan will not have to hand over A. Q. Khan, known as the father of Pakistan's nuclear bomb, to the I.A.E.A. or to any other international authorities for questioning. For two decades, Khan has been linked to a vast consortium of nuclear-black-market activities. Last year,

Musharraf professed to be shocked when Khan, in the face of overwhelming evidence, "confessed" to his activities. A few days later, Musharraf pardoned him, and so far he has refused to allow the I.A.E.A. or American intelligence to interview him. Khan is now said to be living under house arrest in a villa in Islamabad. "It's a deal—a trade-off," the former high-level intelligence official explained. "'Tell us what you know about Iran and we will let your A. Q. Khan guys go.' It's the neoconservatives' version of short-term gain at long-term cost. They want to prove that Bush is the anti-terrorism guy who can handle Iran and the nuclear threat, against the long-term goal of eliminating the black market for nuclear proliferation."

The agreement comes at a time when Musharraf, according to a former high-level Pakistani diplomat, has authorized the expansion of Pakistan's nuclear-weapons arsenal. "Pakistan still needs parts and supplies, and needs to buy them in the clandestine market," the former diplomat said. "The U.S. has done nothing to stop it."

There has also been close, and largely unacknowledged, coöperation with Israel. The government consultant with ties to the Pentagon said that the Defense Department civilians, under the leadership of Douglas Feith, have been working with Israeli planners and consultants to develop and refine potential nuclear, chemical-weapons, and missile targets inside Iran. (After Osirak, Iran situated many of its nuclear sites in remote areas of the east, in an attempt to keep them out of striking range of other countries, especially Israel. Distance no longer lends such protection, however: Israel has acquired three submarines capable of launching cruise missiles and has equipped some of its aircraft with additional fuel tanks, putting Israeli F-16I fighters within the range of most Iranian targets.)

"They believe that about three-quarters of the potential targets can be destroyed from the air, and a quarter are too close to population centers, or buried too deep, to be targeted," the consultant said. Inevitably, he added, some suspicious sites need to be checked out by American or Israeli commando teams—in on-the-ground surveillance—before being targeted.

The Pentagon's contingency plans for a broader invasion of Iran are also being updated. Strategists at the headquarters of the U.S. Central Command, in Tampa, Florida, have been asked to revise the military's war plan, providing for a maximum ground and air invasion of Iran. Updating the plan makes sense, whether or not the Administration intends to act, because the geopolitics of the region have changed dramatically in the last three years. Previously, an American invasion force would have had to enter Iran by sea, by way of the Persian Gulf or the Gulf of Oman; now troops could move in on the ground, from Afghanistan or Iraq. Commando units and other assets could be introduced through new bases in the Central Asian republics.

It is possible that some of the American officials who talk about the need to eliminate Iran's nuclear infrastructure are doing so as part of a propaganda campaign aimed at pressuring Iran to give up its weapons planning. If so, the signals are not always clear. President Bush, who after 9/11 famously depicted Iran as a member of the "axis of evil," is now publicly emphasizing the need for diplomacy to run its course. "We don't have much leverage with the Iranians right now," the President said at a news conference late last year. "Diplomacy must be the first choice, and always the first choice of an administration trying to solve an issue of . . . nuclear armament. And we'll continue to press on diplomacy."

In my interviews over the past two months, I was given a much harsher view. The hawks in the Administration believe that it will soon become clear that the Europeans' negotiated approach cannot succeed, and that at that time the Administration will act. "We're not dealing with a set of National Security Council option papers here," the former high-level intelligence official told me. "They've already passed that wicket. It's not if we're going to do anything against Iran. They're doing it."

The immediate goals of the attacks would be to destroy, or at least temporarily derail, Iran's ability to go nuclear. But there are other, equally purposeful, motives at work. The government consultant told me that the hawks in the Pentagon, in private discussions, have been urging a limited attack on Iran because they believe it could lead to a toppling of the religious leadership. "Within the soul of Iran there is a struggle between secular nationalists and reformers, on the one hand, and, on the other hand, the fundamentalist Islamic movement," the consultant told me. "The minute the aura of invincibility which the mullahs enjoy is shattered, and with it the ability to hoodwink the West, the Iranian regime will collapse"— like the former Communist regimes in Romania, East Germany, and the Soviet Union. Rumsfeld and Wolfowitz share that belief, he said.

"The idea that an American attack on Iran's nuclear facilities would produce a popular uprising is extremely illinformed," said Flynt Leverett, a Middle East scholar who worked on the National Security Council in the Bush Administration. "You have to understand that the nuclear ambition in Iran is supported across the political spectrum, and Iranians will perceive attacks on these sites as attacks on their ambitions to be a major regional player and a modern nation that's technologically sophisticated." Leverett, who is now a senior fellow at the Saban Center for Middle East Policy, at the Brookings Institution, warned that an American attack, if it takes place, "will produce an Iranian backlash against the United States and a rallying around the regime."

Rumsfeld planned and lobbied for more than two years before getting Presidential authority, in a series of findings and executive orders, to use military commandos for covert operations. One of his first steps was bureaucratic: to shift control of an undercover unit, known then as the Gray Fox (it has recently been given a new code name), from the Army to the Special Operations Command (socom), in Tampa. Gray Fox was formally assigned to socom in July, 2002, at the instigation of Rumsfeld's office, which meant that the undercover unit would have a single commander for administration and operational deployment. Then, last fall, Rumsfeld's ability to deploy the commandos expanded. According to a Pentagon consultant, an Execute Order on the Global War on Terrorism (referred to throughout the government as gwot) was issued at Rumsfeld's direction. The order specifically authorized the military "to find and finish" terrorist targets, the consultant said. It included a target list that cited Al Qaeda network members, Al Qaeda senior leadership, and other high-value targets. The consultant said that the order had been cleared throughout the national-security bureaucracy in Washington.

In late November, 2004, the Times reported that Bush had set up an interagency group to study whether it "would best serve the nation" to give the Pentagon complete control over the C.I.A.'s own élite paramilitary unit, which has operated covertly in trouble spots around the world for decades. The panel's conclusions, due in February, are foregone, in the view of many former C.I.A. officers. "It seems like it's going to happen," Howard Hart, who was chief of the C.I.A.'s Paramilitary Operations Division before retiring in 1991, told me.

There was other evidence of Pentagon encroachment. Two former C.I.A. clandestine officers, Vince Cannistraro and Philip Giraldi, who publish Intelligence Brief, a newsletter for their business clients, reported last month on the existence of a broad counter-terrorism Presidential finding that permitted the Pentagon "to operate unilaterally in a number of countries where there is a perception of a clear and evident terrorist threat. . . . A number of the countries are friendly to the U.S. and are major trading partners. Most have been cooperating in the war on terrorism." The two former officers listed some of the countries—Algeria, Sudan, Yemen, Syria, and Malaysia. (I was subsequently told by the former high-level intelligence official that Tunisia is also on the list.)

Giraldi, who served three years in military intelligence before joining the C.I.A., said that he was troubled by the military's expanded covert assignment. "I don't think they can handle the cover," he told me. "They've got to have a different mind-set. They've got to handle new roles and get into foreign cultures and learn how other people think. If you're going into a village and shooting people, it doesn't matter," Giraldi added. "But if you're running operations that involve finesse and sensitivity, the military can't do it. Which is why these kind of operations were always run out of the agency." I was told that many Special Operations officers also have serious misgivings.

Rumsfeld and two of his key deputies, Stephen Cambone, the Under-secretary of Defense for Intelligence, and Army Lieutenant General William G. (Jerry) Boykin, will be part of the chain of command for the new commando operations. Relevant members of the House and Senate intelligence committees have been briefed on the Defense Department's expanded role in covert affairs, a Pentagon adviser assured me, but he did not know how extensive the briefings had been.

"I'm conflicted about the idea of operating without congressional oversight," the Pentagon adviser said. "But I've been told that there will be oversight down to the specific operation." A second Pentagon adviser agreed, with a significant caveat. "There are reporting requirements," he said. "But to execute the finding we don't have to go back and say, 'We're going here and there.' No nitty-gritty detail and no micromanagement."

The legal questions about the Pentagon's right to conduct covert operations without informing Congress have not been resolved. "It's a very, very gray area," said Jeffrey H. Smith, a West Point graduate who served as the C.I.A.'s general counsel in the mid-nineteen-nineties. "Congress believes it voted to include all such covert activities carried out by the armed forces. The military says, 'No, the things we're doing are not intelligence actions under the statute but necessary military steps authorized by the President, as Commander-in-Chief, to "prepare the battlefield."'" Referring to his days at the C.I.A., Smith added, "We were always careful not to use the armed forces in a covert action without a Presidential finding. The Bush Administration has taken a much more aggressive stance."

In his conversation with me, Smith emphasized that he was unaware of the military's current plans for expanding covert action. But he said, "Congress has always worried that the Pentagon is going to get us involved in some military misadventure that nobody knows about."

Under Rumsfeld's new approach, I was told, U.S. military operatives would be permitted to pose abroad as corrupt foreign businessmen seeking to buy contraband items that could be used in nuclear-weapons systems. In some cases, according to the Pentagon advisers, local citizens could be recruited and asked to join up with guerrillas or terrorists. This could potentially involve organizing and carrying out combat operations, or even terrorist activities. Some operations will likely take place in nations in which there is an American diplomatic mission, with an Ambassador and a C.I.A. station chief, the Pentagon consultant said. The Ambassador and the station chief would not necessarily have a need to know, under the Pentagon's current interpretation of its reporting requirement.

The new rules will enable the Special Forces community to set up what it calls "action teams" in the target countries overseas which can be used to find and eliminate terrorist organizations. "Do you remember the right-wing execution squads in El Salvador?" the former high-level intelligence official asked me, referring to the military-led gangs that committed atrocities in the early nineteen-eighties. "We founded them and we financed them," he said. "The objective now is to recruit locals in any area we want. And we aren't going to tell Congress about it." A former military officer, who has knowledge of the Pentagon's commando capabilities, said, "We're going to be riding with the bad boys."

One of the rationales for such tactics was spelled out in a series of articles by John Arquilla, a professor of defense analysis at the Naval Postgraduate School, in Monterey, California, and a consultant on terrorism for the rand corporation. "It takes a network to fight a network," Arquilla wrote in a recent article in the San Francisco Chronicle:

When conventional military operations and bombing failed to defeat the Mau Mau insurgency in Kenya in the 1950s, the British formed teams of friendly Kikuyu tribesmen who went about pretending to be terrorists. These "pseudo gangs," as they were called, swiftly threw the Mau Mau on the defensive, either by befriending and then ambushing bands of fighters or by guiding bombers to the terrorists' camps. What worked in Kenya a half-century ago has a wonderful chance of undermining trust and recruitment among today's terror networks. Forming new pseudo gangs should not be difficult.

"If a confused young man from Marin County can join up with Al Qaeda," Arquilla wrote, referring to John Walker Lindh, the twenty-year-old Californian who was seized in Afghanistan, "think what professional operatives might do."

A few pilot covert operations were conducted last year, one Pentagon adviser told me, and a terrorist cell in Algeria was "rolled up" with American help. The adviser was referring, apparently, to the capture of Ammari Saifi, known as Abderrezak le Para, the head of a North African terrorist network affiliated with Al Qaeda. But at the end of the year there was no agreement within the Defense Department about the rules of engagement. "The issue is approval for the final authority," the former high-level intelligence official said. "Who gets to say 'Get this' or 'Do this'?"

A retired four-star general said, "The basic concept has always been solid, but how do you insure that the people doing it operate within the concept of the law? This is pushing the edge of the envelope." The general added, "It's the oversight. And you're not going to get Warner"—John Warner, of Virginia, the chairman of the Senate Armed Services Committee—"and those guys to exercise oversight. This whole thing goes to the Fourth Deck." He was referring to the floor in the Pentagon where Rumsfeld and Cambone have their offices.

"It's a finesse to give power to Rumsfeld—giving him the right to act swiftly, decisively, and lethally," the first Pentagon adviser told me. "It's a global free-fire zone."

The Pentagon has tried to work around the limits on covert activities before. In the early nineteen-eighties, a covert Army unit was set up and authorized to operate overseas with minimal oversight. The results were disastrous. The Special Operations program was initially known as Intelligence Support Activity, or I.S.A., and was administered from a base near Washington (as was, later, Gray Fox). It was established soon after the failed rescue, in April, 1980, of the American hostages in Iran, who were being held by revolutionary students after the Islamic overthrow of the Shah's regime. At first, the unit was kept secret from many of the senior generals and civilian leaders in the Pentagon, as well as from many members of Congress. It was eventually deployed in the Reagan Administration's war against the Sandinista government, in Nicaragua. It was heavily committed to supporting the Contras. By the mid-eighties, however, the I.S.A.'s operations had been curtailed, and several of its senior officers were courtmartialled following a series of financial scandals, some involving arms deals. The affair was known as "the Yellow Fruit scandal," after the code name given to one of the I.S.A.'s cover organizations—and in many ways the group's procedures laid the groundwork for the Iran-Contra scandal.

Despite the controversy surrounding Yellow Fruit, the I.S.A. was kept intact as an undercover unit by the Army. "But we put so many restrictions on it," the second Pentagon adviser said. "In I.S.A., if you wanted to travel fifty miles you had to get a special order. And there were certain areas, such as Lebanon, where they could not go." The adviser acknowledged that the current operations are similar to those two decades earlier, with similar risks—and, as he saw it, similar reasons for taking the risks. "What drove them then, in terms of Yellow Fruit, was that they had no intelligence on Iran," the adviser told me. "They had no knowledge of Tehran and no people on the ground who could prepare the battle space."

Rumsfeld's decision to revive this approach stemmed, once again, from a failure of intelligence in the Middle East, the adviser said. The Administration believed that the C.I.A. was unable, or unwilling, to provide the military with the information it needed to effectively challenge stateless terrorism. "One of the big challenges was that we didn't have Humint"—human intelligence—"collection capabilities in areas where terrorists existed," the adviser told me. "Because the C.I.A. claimed to have such a hold on Humint, the way to get around them, rather than take them on, was to claim that the agency didn't do Humint to support Special Forces operations overseas. The C.I.A. fought it." Referring to Rumsfeld's new authority for covert operations, the first Pentagon adviser told me, "It's not empowering military intelligence. It's emasculating the C.I.A."

A former senior C.I.A. officer depicted the agency's eclipse as predictable. "For years, the agency bent over backward to integrate and coördinate with the Pentagon," the former officer said. "We just caved and caved and got what we deserved. It is a fact of life today that the Pentagon is a five-hundred-pound gorilla and the C.I.A. director is a chimpanzee."

There was pressure from the White House, too. A former C.I.A. clandestine-services officer told me that, in the months after the resignation of the agency's director George Tenet, in June, 2004, the White House began "coming down critically" on analysts in the C.I.A.'s Directorate of Intelligence (D.I.) and demanded "to see more support for the Administration's political position." Porter Goss, Tenet's successor, engaged in what the recently retired C.I.A. official described as a "political purge" in the D.I. Among the targets were a few senior analysts who were known to write dissenting papers that had been forwarded to the White House. The recently retired C.I.A. official said, "The White House carefully reviewed the political analyses of the D.I. so they could sort out the apostates from the true believers." Some senior analysts in the D.I. have turned in their resignations—quietly, and without revealing the extent of the disarray.

The White House solidified its control over intelligence last month, when it forced last-minute changes in the intelligence-reform bill. The legislation, based substantially on recommendations of the 9/11 Commission, originally gave broad powers, including authority over intelligence spending, to a new national-intelligence director. (The Pentagon controls roughly eighty per cent of the intelligence budget.) A reform bill passed in the Senate by a vote of 96-2. Before the House voted, however, Bush, Cheney, and Rumsfeld balked. The White House publicly supported the legislation, but House Speaker Dennis Hastert refused to bring a House version of the bill to the floor for a vote—ostensibly in defiance of the President, though it was widely understood in Congress that Hastert had been delegated to stall the bill. After intense White House and Pentagon lobbying, the legislation was rewritten. The bill that Congress approved sharply reduced the new director's power, in the name of permitting the Secretary of Defense to maintain his "statutory responsibilities." Fred Kaplan, in the online magazine Slate, described the real issues behind Hastert's action, quoting a congressional aide who expressed amazement as White House lobbyists bashed the Senate bill and came up "with all sorts of ludicrous reasons why it was unacceptable."

"Rummy's plan was to get a compromise in the bill in which the Pentagon keeps its marbles and the C.I.A. loses theirs," the former high-level intelligence official told me. "Then all the pieces of the puzzle fall in place. He gets authority for covert action that is not attributable, the ability to directly task national-intelligence assets"—including the many intelligence satellites that constantly orbit the world.

"Rumsfeld will no longer have to refer anything through the government's intelligence wringer," the former official went on. "The intelligence system was designed to put competing agencies in competition. What's missing will be the dynamic tension that insures everyone's priorities—in the C.I.A., the D.O.D., the F.B.I., and even the Department of Homeland Security—are discussed. The most insidious implication of the new system is that Rumsfeld no longer has to tell people what he's doing so they can ask, 'Why are you doing this?' or 'What are your priorities?' Now he can keep all of the mattress mice out of it."

Writing the Political Past

1.d. From the *Leviathan*

by Thomas Hobbes

> *Readers should try to take a time machine back to Restoration England in the seventeenth century. Thomas Hobbes (1588-1679) believes that monarchy is the most sensible form of government, and he writes in his book that man is a selfish, greedy animal, engaged in unending warfare, which makes the life of man "solitary, poor, nasty, brutish, and short."*

Writers should challenge themselves to read and understand Hobbes' political position in the selected chapters:

- Research Hobbes' biography.

- Do you think the times Hobbes lived in influenced his writings? In what way?

- Do any of Hobbes' social and political thoughts live on in the twenty-first century?

- What would Hobbes say about the war in Iraq?

- What challenges you the most about his language? The text?

Chapter XIII:

Of the Natural Condition of Mankind as Concerning their Felicity and Misery

Nature hath made men so equal in the faculties of body and mind as that, though there be found one man sometimes manifestly stronger in body or of quicker mind than another, yet when all is reckoned together the difference between man and man is not so considerable as that one man can thereupon claim to himself any benefit to which another may not pretend as well as he. For as to the strength of body, the weakest has strength enough to kill the strongest, either by secret machination or by confederacy with others that are in the same danger with himself.

And as to the faculties of the mind, setting aside the arts grounded upon words, and especially that skill of proceeding upon general and infallible rules, called science, which very few have and but in few things, as being not a native faculty born with us, nor attained, as prudence, while we look after somewhat else, I find yet a greater equality amongst men than that of strength. For prudence is but experience, which equal time equally bestows on all men in those things they equally apply themselves unto. That which may perhaps make such equality incredible is but a vain conceit of one's own wisdom, which almost all men think they have in a greater degree than the vulgar; that is, than all men but themselves, and a few others, whom by fame, or for concurring with themselves, they approve. For such is the nature of men that howsoever they may acknowledge many others to be more witty, or more eloquent or more learned, yet they will hardly believe there be many so wise as themselves; for they see their own wit at hand, and other men's at a distance. But this proveth rather that men are in that point equal, than unequal. For there is not ordinarily a greater sign of the equal distribution of anything than that every man is contented with his share.

From this equality of ability ariseth equality of hope in the attaining of our ends. And therefore if any two men desire the same thing, which nevertheless they cannot both enjoy, they become enemies; and in the way to their end (which is principally their own conservation, and sometimes their delectation only) endeavour to destroy or subdue one another. And from hence it comes to pass that where an invader hath no more to fear than another man's single power, if one plant, sow, build, or possess a convenient seat, others may probably be expected to come prepared with forces united to dispossess and deprive him, not only of the fruit of his labour, but also of his life or liberty. And the invader again is in the like danger of another.

And from this diffidence of one another, there is no way for any man to secure himself so reasonable as anticipation; that is, by force, or wiles, to master the persons of all men he can so long till he see no other power great enough to endanger him: and this is no more than his own conservation requireth, and is generally allowed. Also, because there be some that, taking pleasure in contemplating their own power in the acts of conquest, which they pursue farther than their security requires, if others, that otherwise would be glad to be at ease within modest bounds, should not by invasion increase their power, they would not be able, long time, by standing only on their defence, to subsist. And by consequence, such augmentation of dominion over men being necessary to a man's conservation, it ought to be allowed him.

Again, men have no pleasure (but on the contrary a great deal of grief) in keeping company where there is no power able to overawe them all. For every man looketh that his companion should value him at the same rate he sets upon himself, and upon all signs of contempt or undervaluing naturally endeavours, as far as he dares (which amongst them that have no common power to keep them in quiet is far enough to make them destroy each other), to extort a greater value from his contemners, by damage; and from others, by the example.

So that in the nature of man, we find three principal causes of quarrel. First, competition; secondly, diffidence; thirdly, glory. The first maketh men invade for gain; the second, for safety; and the third, for reputation. The first use violence, to make themselves masters of other men's persons, wives, children, and cattle; the second, to defend them; the third, for trifles, as a word, a smile, a different opinion, and any other sign of undervalue, either direct in their persons or by reflection in their kindred, their friends, their nation, their profession, or their name.

Hereby it is manifest that during the time men live without a common power to keep them all in awe, they are in that condition which is called war; and such a war as is of every man against every man. For war consisteth not in battle only, or the act of fighting, but in a tract of time, wherein the will to contend by battle is sufficiently known: and therefore the notion of time is to be considered in the nature of war, as it is in the nature of weather. For as the nature of foul weather lieth not in a shower or two of rain, but in an inclination thereto of many days together: so the nature of war consisteth not in actual fighting, but in the known disposition thereto during all the time there is no assurance to the contrary. All other time is peace.

Whatsoever therefore is consequent to a time of war, where every man is enemy to every man, the same consequent to the time wherein men live without other security than what their own strength and their own invention shall furnish them withal. In such condition there is no place for industry, because the fruit thereof is uncertain: and consequently no culture of the earth; no navigation, nor use of the commodities that may be imported by sea; no commodious building; no instruments of moving and removing such things as require much force; no knowledge of the face of the earth; no account of time; no arts; no letters; no society; and which is worst of all, continual fear, and danger of violent death; and the life of man, solitary, poor, nasty, brutish, and short.

It may seem strange to some man that has not well weighed these things that Nature should thus dissociate and render men apt to invade and destroy one another: and he may therefore, not trusting to this inference, made from the passions, desire perhaps to have the same confirmed by experience. Let him therefore consider with himself: when taking a journey, he arms himself and seeks to go well accompanied; when going to sleep, he locks his doors; when even in his house he locks his chests; and this when he knows there be laws and public officers, armed, to revenge all injuries shall be done him; what opinion he has of his fellow subjects, when he rides armed; of his fellow citizens, when he locks his doors; and of his children, and servants, when he locks his chests. Does he not there as much accuse mankind by his actions as I do by my words? But neither of us accuse man's nature in it. The desires, and other passions of man, are in themselves no sin. No more are the actions that proceed from those passions till they know a law that forbids them; which till laws be made they cannot know, nor can any law be made till they have agreed upon the person that shall make it.

It may peradventure be thought there was never such a time nor condition of war as this; and I believe it was never generally so, over all the world: but there are many places where they live so now. For the savage people in many places of America, except the government of small families, the concord whereof dependeth on natural lust, have no government at all, and live at this day in that brutish manner, as I said before. Howsoever, it may be perceived what manner of life there would be, where there were no common power to fear, by the manner of life which men that have formerly lived under a peaceful government use to degenerate into a civil war.

But though there had never been any time wherein particular men were in a condition of war one against another, yet in all times kings and persons of sovereign authority, because of their independency, are in continual jealousies, and in the state and posture of gladiators, having their weapons pointing, and their eyes fixed on one another; that is, their forts, garrisons, and guns upon the frontiers of their kingdoms, and continual spies upon their neighbours, which is a posture of war. But because they uphold thereby the industry of their subjects, there does not follow from it that misery which accompanies the liberty of particular men.

To this war of every man against every man, this also is consequent; that nothing can be unjust. The notions of right and wrong, justice and injustice, have there no place. Where there is no common power, there is no law; where no law, no injustice. Force and fraud are in war the two cardinal virtues. Justice and injustice are none of the faculties neither of the body nor mind. If they were, they might be in a man that were alone in the world, as well as his senses and passions. They are qualities that relate to men in society, not in solitude. It is consequent also to the same condition that there be no propriety, no dominion, no mine and thine distinct; but only that to be every man's that he can get, and for so long as he can keep it. And thus much for the ill condition which man by mere nature is actually placed in; though with a possibility to come out of it, consisting partly in the passions, partly in his reason.

The passions that incline men to peace are: fear of death; desire of such things as are necessary to commodious living; and a hope by their industry to obtain them. And reason suggesteth convenient articles of peace upon which men may be drawn to agreement. These articles are they which otherwise are called the laws of nature, whereof I shall speak more particularly in the two following chapters.

CHAPTER XIV:
Of the First and Second Natural Laws, and of Contracts

The right of nature, which writers commonly call jus naturale, is the liberty each man hath to use his own power as he will himself for the preservation of his own nature; that is to say, of his own life; and consequently, of doing anything which, in his own judgement and reason, he shall conceive to be the aptest means thereunto.

By liberty is understood, according to the proper signification of the word, the absence of external impediments; which impediments may oft take away part of a man's power to do what he would, but cannot hinder him from using the power left him according as his judgement and reason shall dictate to him.

A law of nature, lex naturalis, is a precept, or general rule, found out by reason, by which a man is forbidden to do that which is destructive of his life, or taketh away the means of preserving the same, and to omit that by which he thinketh it may be best preserved. For though they that speak of this subject use to confound jus and lex, right and law, yet they ought to be distinguished, because right consisteth in liberty to do, or to forbear; whereas law determineth and bindeth to one of them: so that law and right differ as much as obligation and liberty, which in one and the same matter are inconsistent.

And because the condition of man (as hath been declared in the precedent chapter) is a condition of war of every one against every one, in which case every one is governed by his own reason, and there is nothing he can make use of that may not be a help unto him in preserving his life against his enemies; it followeth that in such a condition every man has a right to every thing, even to one another's body. And therefore, as long as this natural right of every man to every thing endureth, there can be no security to any man, how strong or wise soever he be, of living out the time which nature ordinarily alloweth men to live. And consequently it is a precept, or general rule of reason: that every man ought to endeavour peace, as far as he has hope of obtaining it; and when he cannot obtain it, that he may seek and use all helps and advantages of war. The first branch of which rule containeth the first and fundamental law of nature, which is: to seek peace and follow it. The second, the sum of the right of nature, which is: by all means we can to defend ourselves.

From this fundamental law of nature, by which men are commanded to endeavour peace, is derived this second law: that a man be willing, when others are so too, as far forth as for peace and defence of himself he shall think it necessary, to lay down this right to all things; and be contented with so much liberty against other men as he would allow other men against himself. For as long as every man holdeth this right, of doing anything he liketh; so long are all men in the condition of war. But if other men will not lay down their right, as well as he, then there is no reason for anyone to divest himself of his: for that were to expose himself to prey, which no man is bound to, rather than to dispose himself to peace. This is that law of the gospel: Whatsoever you require that others should do to you, that do ye to them. And that law of all men, quod tibi fieri non vis, alteri ne feceris.

To lay down a man's right to anything is to divest himself of the liberty of hindering another of the benefit of his own right to the same. For he that renounceth or passeth away his right giveth not to any other man a right which he had not before, because there is nothing to which every man had not right by nature, but only standeth out of his way that he may enjoy his own original right without hindrance from him, not without hindrance from another. So that the effect which redoundeth to one man by another man's defect of right is but so much diminution of impediments to the use of his own right original.

Right is laid aside, either by simply renouncing it, or by transferring it to another. By simply renouncing, when he cares not to whom the benefit thereof redoundeth. By transferring, when he intendeth the benefit thereof to some certain person or persons. And when a man hath in either manner abandoned or granted away his right, then is he said to be obliged, or bound, not to hinder those to whom such right is granted, or abandoned, from the benefit of it: and that he ought, and it is duty, not to make void that voluntary act of his own: and that such hindrance is injustice, and injury, as being sine jure; the right being before renounced or transferred. So that injury or injustice, in the controversies of the world, is somewhat like to that which in the disputations of scholars is called absurdity. For as it is there called an absurdity to contradict what one maintained in the beginning; so in the world it is called injustice, and injury voluntarily to undo that which from the beginning he had voluntarily done. The way by which a man either simply renounceth or transferreth his right is a declaration, or signification, by some voluntary and sufficient sign, or signs, that he doth so renounce or transfer, or hath so renounced or transferred the same, to him that accepteth it. And these signs are either words only, or actions only; or, as it happeneth most often, both words and actions. And the same are the bonds, by which men are bound and obliged: bonds that have their strength, not from their own nature (for nothing is more easily broken than a man's word), but from fear of some evil consequence upon the rupture.

Whensoever a man transferreth his right, or renounceth it, it is either in consideration of some right reciprocally transferred to himself, or for some other good he hopeth for thereby. For it is a voluntary act: and of the voluntary acts of every man, the object is some good to himself. And therefore there be some rights which no man can be understood by any words, or other signs, to have abandoned or transferred. As first a man cannot lay down the right of resisting them that assault him by force to take away his life, because he cannot be understood to aim thereby at any good to himself. The same may be said of wounds, and chains, and imprisonment, both because there is no benefit consequent to such patience, as there is to the patience of suffering another to be wounded or imprisoned, as also because a man cannot tell when he seeth men proceed against him by violence whether they intend his death or not. And lastly the motive and end for which this renouncing and transferring of right is introduced is nothing else but the security of a man's person, in his life, and in the means of so preserving life as not to be weary of it. And therefore if a man by words, or other signs, seem to despoil himself of the end for which those signs were intended, he is not to be understood as if he meant it, or that it was his will, but that he was ignorant of how such words and actions were to be interpreted.

The mutual transferring of right is that which men call contract.

There is difference between transferring of right to the thing, the thing, and transferring or tradition, that is, delivery of the thing itself. For the thing may be delivered together with the translation of the right, as in buying and selling with ready money, or exchange of goods or lands, and it may be delivered some time after.

Again, one of the contractors may deliver the thing contracted for on his part, and leave the other to perform his part at some determinate time after, and in the meantime be trusted; and then the contract on his part is called pact, or covenant: or both parts may contract now to perform hereafter, in which cases he that is to perform in time to come, being trusted, his performance is called keeping of promise, or faith, and the failing of performance, if it be voluntary, violation of faith.

When the transferring of right is not mutual, but one of the parties transferreth in hope to gain thereby friendship or service from another, or from his friends; or in hope to gain the reputation of charity, or magnanimity; or to deliver his mind from the pain of compassion; or in hope of reward in heaven; this is not contract, but gift, free gift, grace: which words signify one and the same thing.

Signs of contract are either express or by inference. Express are words spoken with understanding of what they signify: and such words are either of the time present or past; as, I give, I grant, I have given, I have granted, I will that this be yours: or of the future; as, I will give, I will grant, which words of the future are called promise.

Signs by inference are sometimes the consequence of words; sometimes the consequence of silence; sometimes the consequence of actions; sometimes the consequence of forbearing an action: and generally a sign by inference, of any contract, is whatsoever sufficiently argues the will of the contractor.

Words alone, if they be of the time to come, and contain a bare promise, are an insufficient sign of a free gift and therefore not obligatory. For if they be of the time to come, as, tomorrow I will give, they are a sign I have not given yet, and consequently that my right is not transferred, but remaineth till I transfer it by some other act. But if the words be of the time present, or past, as, I have given, or do give to be delivered tomorrow, then is my tomorrow's right given away today; and that by the virtue of the words, though there were no other argument of my will. And there is a great difference in the signification of these words, volo hoc tuum esse cras, and cras dabo; that is, between I will that this be thine tomorrow, and, I will give it thee tomorrow: for the word I will, in the former manner of speech, signifies an act of the will present; but in the latter, it signifies a promise of an act of the will to come: and therefore the former words, being of the present, transfer a future right; the latter, that be of the future, transfer nothing. But if there be other signs of the will to transfer a right besides words; then, though the gift be free, yet may the right be understood to pass by words of the future: as if a man propound a prize to him that comes first to the end of a race, the gift is free; and though the words be of the future, yet the right passeth: for if he would not have his words so be understood, he should not have let them run.

In contracts the right passeth, not only where the words are of the time present or past, but also where they are of the future, because all contract is mutual translation, or change of right; and therefore he that promiseth only, because he hath already received the benefit for which he promiseth, is to be understood as if he intended the right should pass: for unless he had been content to have his words so understood, the other would not have performed his part first. And for that cause, in buying, and selling, and other acts of contract, a promise is equivalent to a covenant, and therefore obligatory.

He that performeth first in the case of a contract is said to merit that which he is to receive by the performance of the other, and he hath it as due. Also when a prize is propounded to many, which is to be given to him only that winneth, or money is thrown amongst many to be enjoyed by them that catch it; though this be a free gift, yet so to win, or so to catch, is to merit, and to have it as due. For the right is transferred in the propounding of the prize, and in throwing down the money, though it be not determined to whom, but by the event of the contention. But there is between these two sorts of merit this difference, that in contract I merit by virtue of my own power and the contractor's need, but in this case of free gift I am enabled to merit only by the benignity of the giver: in contract I merit at the contractor's hand that he should depart with his right; in this case of gift, I merit not that the giver should part with his right, but that when he has parted with it, it should be mine rather than another's. And this I think to be the meaning of that distinction of the Schools between meritum congrui and meritum condigni. For God Almighty, having promised paradise to those men, hoodwinked with carnal desires, that can walk through this world according to the precepts and limits prescribed by him, they say he that shall so walk shall merit paradise ex congruo.

But because no man can demand a right to it by his own righteousness, or any other power in himself, but by the free grace of God only, they say no man can merit paradise ex condigno. This, I say, I think is the meaning of that distinction; but because disputers do not agree upon the signification of their own terms of art longer than it serves their turn, I will not affirm anything of their meaning: only this I say; when a gift is given indefinitely, as a prize to be contended for, he that winneth meriteth, and may claim the prize as due.

If a covenant be made wherein neither of the parties perform presently, but trust one another, in the condition of mere nature (which is a condition of war of every man against every man) upon any reasonable suspicion, it is void: but if there be a common power set over them both, with right and force sufficient to compel performance, it is not void. For he that performeth first has no assurance the other will perform after, because the bonds of words are too weak to bridle men's ambition, avarice, anger, and other passions, without the fear of some coercive power; which in the condition of mere nature, where all men are equal, and judges of the justness of their own fears, cannot possibly be supposed. And therefore he which performeth first does but betray himself to his enemy, contrary to the right he can never abandon of defending his life and means of living.

But in a civil estate, where there a power set up to constrain those that would otherwise violate their faith, that fear is no more reasonable; and for that cause, he which by the covenant is to perform first is obliged so to do.

The cause of fear, which maketh such a covenant invalid, must be always something arising after the covenant made, as some new fact or other sign of the will not to perform, else it cannot make the covenant void. For that which could not hinder a man from promising ought not to be admitted as a hindrance of performing.

He that transferreth any right transferreth the means of enjoying it, as far as lieth in his power. As he that selleth land is understood to transfer the herbage and whatsoever grows upon it; nor can he that sells a mill turn away the stream that drives it. And they that give to a man the right of government in sovereignty are understood to give him the right of levying money to maintain soldiers, and of appointing magistrates for the administration of justice.

To make covenants with brute beasts is impossible, because not understanding our speech, they understand not, nor accept of any translation of right, nor can translate any right to another: and without mutual acceptation, there is no covenant.

To make covenant with God is impossible but by mediation of such as God speaketh to, either by revelation supernatural or by His lieutenants that govern under Him and in His name: for otherwise we know not whether our covenants be accepted or not. And therefore they that vow anything contrary to any law of nature, vow in vain, as being a thing unjust to pay such vow. And if it be a thing commanded by the law of nature, it is not the vow, but the law that binds them.

The matter or subject of a covenant is always something that falleth under deliberation, for to covenant is an act of the will; that is to say, an act, and the last act, of deliberation; and is therefore always understood to be something to come, and which judged possible for him that covenanteth to perform.

And therefore, to promise that which is known to be impossible is no covenant. But if that prove impossible afterwards, which before was thought possible, the covenant is valid and bindeth, though not to the thing itself, yet to the value; or, if that also be impossible, to the unfeigned endeavour of performing as much as is possible, for to more no man can be obliged.

Men are freed of their covenants two ways; by performing, or by being forgiven. For performance is the natural end of obligation, and forgiveness the restitution of liberty, as being a retransferring of that right in which the obligation consisted.

Covenants entered into by fear, in the condition of mere nature, are obligatory. For example, if I covenant to pay a ransom, or service for my life, to an enemy, I am bound by it. For it is a contract, wherein one receiveth the benefit of life; the other is to receive money, or service for it, and consequently, where no other law (as in the condition of mere nature) forbiddeth the performance, the covenant is valid. Therefore prisoners of war, if trusted with the payment of their ransom, are obliged to pay it: and if a weaker prince make a disadvantageous peace with a stronger, for fear, he is bound to keep it; unless (as hath been said before) there ariseth some new and just cause of fear to renew the war. And even in Commonwealths, if I be forced to redeem myself from a thief by promising him money, I am bound to pay it, till the civil law discharge me. For whatsoever I may lawfully do without obligation, the same I may lawfully covenant to do through fear: and what I lawfully covenant, I cannot lawfully break.

A former covenant makes void a later. For a man that hath passed away his right to one man today hath it not to pass tomorrow to another: and therefore the later promise passeth no right, but is null.

A covenant not to defend myself from force, by force, is always void. For (as I have shown before) no man can transfer or lay down his right to save himself from death, wounds, and imprisonment, the avoiding whereof is the only end of laying down any right; and therefore the promise of not resisting force, in no covenant transferreth any right, nor is obliging. For though a man may covenant thus, unless I do so, or so, kill me; he cannot covenant thus, unless I do so, or so, I will not resist you when you come to kill me.

For man by nature chooseth the lesser evil, which is danger of death in resisting, rather than the greater, which is certain and present death in not resisting. And this is granted to be true by all men, in that they lead criminals to execution, and prison, with armed men, notwithstanding that such criminals have consented to the law by which they are condemned.

A covenant to accuse oneself, without assurance of pardon, is likewise invalid. For in the condition of nature where every man is judge, there is no place for accusation: and in the civil state the accusation is followed with punishment, which, being force, a man is not obliged not to resist. The same is also true of the accusation of those by whose condemnation a man falls into misery; as of a father, wife, or benefactor. For the testimony of such an accuser, if it be not willingly given, is presumed to be corrupted by nature, and therefore not to be received: and where a man's testimony is not to be credited, he is not bound to give it. Also accusations upon torture are not to be reputed as testimonies. For torture is to be used but as means of conjecture, and light, in the further examination and search of truth: and what is in that case confessed tendeth to the ease of him that is tortured, not to the informing of the torturers, and therefore ought not to have the credit of a sufficient testimony: for whether he deliver himself by true or false accusation, he does it by the right of preserving his own life.

The force of words being (as I have formerly noted) too weak to hold men to the performance of their covenants, there are in man's nature but two imaginable helps to strengthen it. And those are either a fear of the consequence of breaking their word, or a glory or pride in appearing not to need to break it. This latter is a generosity too rarely found to be presumed on, especially in the pursuers of wealth, command, or sensual pleasure, which are the greatest part of mankind. The passion to be reckoned upon is fear; whereof there be two very general objects: one, the power of spirits invisible; the other, the power of those men they shall therein offend. Of these two, though the former be the greater power, yet the fear of the latter is commonly the greater fear. The fear of the former is in every man his own religion, which hath place in the nature of man before civil society. The latter hath not so; at least not place enough to keep men to their promises, because in the condition of mere nature, the inequality of power is not discerned, but by the event of battle. So that before the time of civil society, or in the interruption thereof by war, there is nothing can strengthen a covenant of peace agreed on against the temptations of avarice, ambition, lust, or other strong desire, but the fear of that invisible power which they every one worship as God, and fear as a revenger of their perfidy. All therefore that can be done between two men not subject to civil power is to put one another to swear by the God he feareth: which swearing, or oath, is a form of speech, added to a promise, by which he that promiseth signifieth that unless he perform he renounceth the mercy of his God, or calleth to him for vengeance on himself. Such was the heathen form, Let Jupiter kill me else, as I kill this beast. So is our form, I shall do thus, and thus, so help me God. And this, with the rites and ceremonies which every one useth in his own religion, that the fear of breaking faith might be the greater.

By this it appears that an oath taken according to any other form, or rite, than his that sweareth is in vain and no oath, and that there is no swearing by anything which the swearer thinks not God. For though men have sometimes used to swear by their kings, for fear, or flattery; yet they would have it thereby understood they attributed to them divine honour. And that swearing unnecessarily by God is but profaning of his name: and swearing by other things, as men do in common discourse, is not swearing, but an impious custom, gotten by too much vehemence of talking.

It appears also that the oath adds nothing to the obligation. For a covenant, if lawful, binds in the sight of God, without the oath, as much as with it; if unlawful, bindeth not at all, though it be confirmed with an oath.

CHAPTER XV:

Of other Laws of Nature

FROM that law of nature by which we are obliged to transfer to another such rights as, being retained, hinder the peace of mankind, there followeth a third; which is this: that men perform their covenants made; without which covenants are in vain, and but empty words; and the right of all men to all things remaining, we are still in the condition of war.

And in this law of nature consisteth the fountain and original of justice. For where no covenant hath preceded, there hath no right been transferred, and every man has right to everything and consequently, no action can be unjust. But when a covenant is made, then to break it is unjust and the definition of injustice is no other than the not performance of covenant. And whatsoever is not unjust is just.

But because covenants of mutual trust, where there is a fear of not performance on either part (as hath been said in the former chapter), are invalid, though the original of justice be the making of covenants, yet injustice actually there can be none till the cause of such fear be taken away; which, while men are in the natural condition of war, cannot be done. Therefore before the names of just and unjust can have place, there must be some coercive power to compel men equally to the performance of their covenants, by the terror of some punishment greater than the benefit they expect by the breach of their covenant, and to make good that propriety which by mutual contract men acquire in recompense of the universal right they abandon: and such power there is none before the erection of a Commonwealth. And this is also to be gathered out of the ordinary definition of justice in the Schools, for they say that justice is the constant will of giving to every man his own. And therefore where there is no own, that is, no propriety, there is no injustice; and where there is no coercive power erected, that is, where there is no Commonwealth, there is no propriety, all men having right to all things: therefore where there is no Commonwealth, there nothing is unjust. So that the nature of justice consisteth in keeping of valid covenants, but the validity of covenants begins not but with the constitution of a civil power sufficient to compel men to keep them: and then it is also that propriety begins.

The fool hath said in his heart, there is no such thing as justice, and sometimes also with his tongue, seriously alleging that every man's conservation and contentment being committed to his own care, there could be no reason why every man might not do what he thought conduced thereunto: and therefore also to make, or not make; keep, or not keep, covenants was not against reason when it conduced to one's benefit. He does not therein deny that there be covenants; and that they are sometimes broken, sometimes kept; and that such breach of them may be called injustice, and the observance of them justice: but he questioneth whether injustice, taking away the fear of God (for the same fool hath said in his heart there is no God), not sometimes stand with that reason which dictateth to every man his own good; and particularly then, when it conduceth to such a benefit as shall put a man in a condition to neglect not only the dispraise and revilings, but also the power of other men. The kingdom of God is gotten by violence: but what if it could be gotten by unjust violence? Were it against reason so to get it, when it is impossible to receive hurt by it? And if it be not against reason, it is not against justice: or else justice is not to be approved for good. From such reasoning as this, successful wickedness hath obtained the name of virtue: and some that in all other things have disallowed the violation of faith, yet have allowed it when it is for the getting of a kingdom. And the heathen that believed that Saturn was deposed by his son Jupiter believed nevertheless the same Jupiter to be the avenger of injustice, somewhat like to a piece of law in Coke's Commentaries on Littleton; where he says if the right heir of the crown be attainted of treason, yet the crown shall descend to him, and eo instante the attainder be void: from which instances a man will be very prone to infer that when the heir apparent of a kingdom shall kill him that is in possession, though his father, you may call it injustice, or by what other name you will; yet it can never be against reason, seeing all the voluntary actions of men tend to the benefit of themselves; and those actions are most reasonable that conduce most to their ends. This specious reasoning is nevertheless false.

For the question is not of promises mutual, where there is no security of performance on either side, as when there is no civil power erected over the parties promising; for such promises are no covenants: but either where one of the parties has performed already, or where there is a power to make him perform, there is the question whether it be against reason; that is, against the benefit of the other to perform, or not. And I say it is not against reason. For the manifestation whereof we are to consider; first, that when a man doth a thing, which notwithstanding anything can be foreseen and reckoned on tendeth to his own destruction, howsoever some accident, which he could not expect, arriving may turn it to his benefit; yet such events do not make it reasonably or wisely done. Secondly, that in a condition of war, wherein every man to every man, for want of a common power to keep them all in awe, is an enemy, there is no man can hope by his own strength, or wit, to himself from destruction without the help of confederates; where every one expects the same defence by the confederation that any one else does: and therefore he which declares he thinks it reason to deceive those that help him can in reason expect no other means of safety than what can be had from his own single power. He, therefore, that breaketh his covenant, and consequently declareth that he thinks he may with reason do so, cannot be received into any society that unite themselves for peace and defence but by the error of them that receive him; nor when he is received be retained in it without seeing the danger of their error; which errors a man cannot reasonably reckon upon as the means of his security: and therefore if he be left, or cast out of society, he perisheth; and if he live in society, it is by the errors of other men, which he could not foresee nor reckon upon, and consequently against the reason of his preservation; and so, as all men that contribute not to his destruction forbear him only out of ignorance of what is good for themselves.

As for the instance of gaining the secure and perpetual felicity of heaven by any way, it is frivolous; there being but one way imaginable, and that is not breaking, but keeping of covenant.

And for the other instance of attaining sovereignty by rebellion; it is manifest that, though the event follow, yet because it cannot reasonably be expected, but rather the contrary, and because by gaining it so, others are taught to gain the same in like manner, the attempt thereof is against reason. Justice therefore, that is to say, keeping of covenant, is a rule of reason by which we are forbidden to do anything destructive to our life, and consequently a law of nature.

There be some that proceed further and will not have the law of nature to be those rules which conduce to the preservation of man's life on earth, but to the attaining of an eternal felicity after death; to which they think the breach of covenant may conduce, and consequently be just and reasonable; such are they that think it a work of merit to kill, or depose, or rebel against the sovereign power constituted over them by their own consent. But because there is no natural knowledge of man's estate after death, much less of the reward that is then to be given to breach of faith, but only a belief grounded upon other men's saying that they know it supernaturally or that they know those that knew them that knew others that knew it supernaturally, breach of faith cannot be called a precept of reason or nature.

Others, that allow for a law of nature the keeping of faith, do nevertheless make exception of certain persons; as heretics, and such as use not to perform their covenant to others; and this also is against reason. For if any fault of a man be sufficient to discharge our covenant made, the same ought in reason to have been sufficient to have hindered the making of it.

The names of just and unjust when they are attributed to men, signify one thing, and when they are attributed to actions, another. When they are attributed to men, they signify conformity, or inconformity of manners, to reason. But when they are attributed to action they signify the conformity, or inconformity to reason, not of manners, or manner of life, but of particular actions. A just man therefore is he that taketh all the care he can that his actions may be all just; and an unjust man is he that neglecteth it. And such men are more often in our language styled by the names of righteous and unrighteous than just and unjust though the meaning be the same. Therefore a righteous man does not lose that title by one or a few unjust actions that proceed from sudden passion, or mistake of things or persons, nor does an unrighteous man lose his character for such actions as he does, or forbears to do, for fear: because his will is not framed by the justice, but by the apparent benefit of what he is to do. That which gives to human actions the relish of justice is a certain nobleness or gallantness of courage, rarely found, by which a man scorns to be beholding for the contentment of his life to fraud, or breach of promise. This justice of the manners is that which is meant where justice is called a virtue; and injustice, a vice.

But the justice of actions denominates men, not just, but guiltless: and the injustice of the same (which is also called injury) gives them but the name of guilty.

Again, the injustice of manners is the disposition or aptitude to do injury, and is injustice before it proceed to act, and without supposing any individual person injured. But the injustice of an action (that is to say, injury) supposeth an individual person injured; namely him to whom the covenant was made: and therefore many times the injury is received by one man when the damage redoundeth to another. As when the master commandeth his servant to give money to stranger; if it be not done, the injury is done to the master, whom he had before covenanted to obey; but the damage redoundeth to the stranger, to whom he had no obligation, and therefore could not injure him. And so also in Commonwealths private men may remit to one another their debts, but not robberies or other violences, whereby they are endamaged; because the detaining of debt is an injury to themselves, but robbery and violence are injuries to the person of the Commonwealth.

Whatsoever is done to a man, conformable to his own will signified to the doer, is not injury to him. For if he that doeth it hath not passed away his original right to do what he please by some antecedent covenant, there is no breach of covenant, and therefore no injury done him. And if he have, then his will to have it done, being signified, is a release of that covenant, and so again there is no injury done him.

Justice of actions is by writers divided into commutative and distributive: and the former they say consisteth in proportion arithmetical; the latter in proportion geometrical. Commutative, therefore, they place in the equality of value of the things contracted for; and distributive, in the distribution of equal benefit to men of equal merit. As if it were injustice to sell dearer than we buy, or to give more to a man than he merits. The value of all things contracted for is measured by the appetite of the contractors, and therefore the just value is that which they be contented to give. And merit (besides that which is by covenant, where the performance on one part meriteth the performance of the other part, and falls under justice commutative, not distributive) is not due by justice, but is rewarded of grace only. And therefore this distinction, in the sense wherein it useth to be expounded, is not right. To speak properly, commutative justice is the justice of a contractor; that is, a performance of covenant in buying and selling, hiring and letting to hire, lending and borrowing, exchanging, bartering, and other acts of contract.

And distributive justice, the justice of an arbitrator; that is to say, the act of defining what is just. Wherein, being trusted by them that make him arbitrator, if he perform his trust, he is said to distribute to every man his own: and this is indeed just distribution, and may be called, though improperly, distributive justice, but more properly equity, which also is a law of nature, as shall be shown in due place.

As justice dependeth on antecedent covenant; so does gratitude depend on antecedent grace; that is to say, antecedent free gift; and is the fourth law of nature, which may be conceived in this form: that a man which receiveth benefit from another of mere grace endeavour that he which giveth it have no reasonable cause to repent him of his good will. For no man giveth but with intention of good to himself, because gift is voluntary; and of all voluntary acts, the object is to every man his own good; of which if men see they shall be frustrated, there will be no beginning of benevolence or trust, nor consequently of mutual help, nor of reconciliation of one man to another; and therefore they are to remain still in the condition of war, which is contrary to the first and fundamental law of nature which commandeth men to seek peace. The breach of this law is called ingratitude, and hath the same relation to grace that injustice hath to obligation by covenant.

A fifth law of nature is complaisance; that is to say, that every man strive to accommodate himself to the rest. For the understanding whereof we may consider that there is in men's aptness to society a diversity of nature, rising from their diversity of affections, not unlike to that we see in stones brought together for building of an edifice. For as that stone which by the asperity and irregularity of figure takes more room from others than itself fills, and for hardness cannot be easily made plain, and thereby hindereth the building, is by the builders cast away as unprofitable and troublesome: so also, a man that by asperity of nature will strive to retain those things which to himself are superfluous, and to others necessary, and for the stubbornness of his passions cannot be corrected, is to be left or cast out of society as cumbersome thereunto. For seeing every man, not only by right, but also by necessity of nature, is supposed to endeavour all he can to obtain that which is necessary for his conservation, he that shall oppose himself against it for things superfluous is guilty of the war that thereupon is to follow, and therefore doth that which is contrary to the fundamental law of nature, which commandeth to seek peace. The observers of this law may be called sociable, (the Latins call them commodi); the contrary, stubborn, insociable, forward, intractable.

A sixth law of nature is this: that upon caution of the future time, a man ought to pardon the offences past of them that, repenting, desire it. For pardon is nothing but granting of peace; which though granted to them that persevere in their hostility, be not peace, but fear; yet not granted to them that give caution of the future time is sign of an aversion to peace, and therefore contrary to the law of nature.

A seventh is: that in revenges (that is, retribution of evil for evil), men look not at the greatness of the evil past, but the greatness of the good to follow. Whereby we are forbidden to inflict punishment with any other design than for correction of the offender, or direction of others. For this law is consequent to the next before it, that commandeth pardon upon security of the future time. Besides, revenge without respect to the example and profit to come is a triumph, or glorying in the hurt of another, tending to no end (for the end is always somewhat to come); and glorying to no end is vain-glory, and contrary to reason; and to hurt without reason tendeth to the introduction of war, which is against the law of nature, and is commonly styled by the name of cruelty.

And because all signs of hatred, or contempt, provoke to fight; insomuch as most men choose rather to hazard their life than not to be revenged, we may in the eighth place, for a law of nature, set down this precept: that no man by deed, word, countenance, or gesture, declare hatred or contempt of another. The breach of which law is commonly called contumely.

The question who is the better man has no place in the condition of mere nature, where (as has been shown before) all men are equal. The inequality that now is has been introduced by the laws civil. I know that Aristotle in the first book of his Politics, for a foundation of his doctrine, maketh men by nature, some more worthy to command, meaning the wiser sort, such as he thought himself to be for his philosophy; others to serve, meaning those that had strong bodies, but were not philosophers as he; as master and servant were not introduced by consent of men, but by difference of wit: which is not only against reason, but also against experience. For there are very few so foolish that had not rather govern themselves than be governed by others: nor when the wise, in their own conceit, contend by force with them who distrust their own wisdom, do they always, or often, or almost at any time, get the victory. If nature therefore have made men equal, that equality is to be acknowledged: or if nature have made men unequal, yet because men that think themselves equal will not enter into conditions of peace, but upon equal terms, such equality must be admitted. And therefore for the ninth law of nature, I put this: that every man acknowledge another for his equal by nature. The breach of this precept is pride.

On this law dependeth another: that at the entrance into conditions of peace, no man require to reserve to himself any right which he is not content should he reserved to every one of the rest. As it is necessary for all men that seek peace to lay down certain rights of nature; that is to say, not to have liberty to do all they list, so is it necessary for man's life to retain some: as right to govern their own bodies;

enjoy air, water, motion, ways to go from place to place; and all things else without which a man cannot live, or not live well. If in this case, at the making of peace, men require for themselves that which they would not have to be granted to others, they do contrary to the precedent law that commandeth the acknowledgement of natural equality, and therefore also against the law of nature. The observers of this law are those we call modest, and the breakers arrogant men. The Greeks call the violation of this law pleonexia; that is, a desire of more than their share.

Also, if a man he trusted to judge between man and man, it is a precept of the law of nature that he deal equally between them. For without that, the controversies of men cannot be determined but by war. He therefore that is partial in judgement, doth what in him lies to deter men from the use of judges and arbitrators, and consequently, against the fundamental law of nature, is the cause of war. The observance of this law, from the equal distribution to each man of that which in reason belonged to him, is called equity, and (as I have said before) distributive justice: the violation, acception of persons, prosopolepsia.

And from this followeth another law: that such things as cannot he divided be enjoyed in common, if it can be; and if the quantity of the thing permit, without stint; otherwise proportionably to the number of them that have right. For otherwise the distribution is unequal, and contrary to equity.

But some things there be that can neither be divided nor enjoyed in common. Then, the law of nature which prescribeth equity requireth: that the entire right, or else (making the use alternate) the first possession, be determined by lot. For equal distribution is of the law of nature; and other means of equal distribution cannot be imagined.

Of lots there be two sorts, arbitrary and natural. Arbitrary is that which is agreed on by the competitors; natural is either primogeniture (which the Greek calls kleronomia, which signifies, given by lot), or first seizure.

And therefore those things which cannot be enjoyed in common, nor divided, ought to be adjudged to the first possessor; and in some cases to the first born, as acquired by lot.

It is also a law of nature: that all men that mediate peace he allowed safe conduct. For the law that commandeth peace, as the end, commandeth intercession, as the means; and to intercession the means is safe conduct.

And because, though men be never so willing to observe these laws, there may nevertheless arise questions concerning a man's action; first, whether it were done, or not done; secondly, if done, whether against the law, or not against the law; the former whereof is called a question of fact, the latter a question of right; therefore unless the parties to the question covenant mutually to stand to the sentence of another, they are as far from peace as ever. This other, to whose sentence they submit, is called an arbitrator. And therefore it is of the law of nature that they that are at controversy submit their right to the judgment of an arbitrator.

And seeing every man is presumed to do all things in order to his own benefit, no man is a fit arbitrator in his own cause: and if he were never so fit, yet equity allowing to each party equal benefit, if one be admitted to be judge, the other is to be admitted also; and so the controversy, that is, the cause of war, remains, against the law of nature.

For the same reason no man in any cause ought to be received for arbitrator to whom greater profit, or honour, or pleasure apparently ariseth out of the victory of one party than of the other: for he hath taken, though an unavoidable bribe, yet a bribe; and no man can be obliged to trust him. And thus also the controversy and the condition of war remaineth, contrary to the law of nature.

And in a controversy of fact, the judge being to give no more credit to one than to the other, if there be no other arguments, must give credit to a third; or to a third and fourth; or more: for else the question is undecided, and left to force, contrary to the law of nature.

These are the laws of nature, dictating peace, for a means of the conservation of men in multitudes; and which only concern the doctrine of civil society. There be other things tending to the destruction of particular men; as drunkenness, and all other parts of intemperance, which may therefore also be reckoned amongst those things which the law of nature hath forbidden, but are not necessary to be mentioned, nor are pertinent enough to this place.

And though this may seem too subtle a deduction of the laws of nature to be taken notice of by all men, whereof the most part are too busy in getting food, and the rest too negligent to understand; yet to leave all men inexcusable, they have been contracted into one easy sum, intelligible even to the meanest capacity; and that is: Do not that to another which thou wouldest not have done to thyself, which showeth him that he has no more to do in learning the laws of nature but, when weighing the actions of other men with his own they seem too heavy, to put them into the other part of the balance, and his own into their place, that his own passions and self-love may add nothing to the weight; and then there is none of these laws of nature that will not appear unto him very reasonable.

The laws of nature oblige in foro interno; that is to say, they bind to a desire they should take place: but in foro externo; that is, to the putting them in act, not always. For he that should be modest and tractable, and perform all he promises in such time and place where no man else should do so, should but make himself a prey to others, and procure his own certain ruin, contrary to the ground of all laws of nature which tend to nature's preservation. And again, he that having sufficient security that others shall observe the same laws towards him, observes them not himself, seeketh not peace, but war, and consequently the destruction of his nature by violence.

And whatsoever laws bind in foro interno may be broken, not only by a fact contrary to the law, but also by a fact according to it, in case a man think it contrary. For though his action in this case be according to the law, yet his purpose was against the law; which, where the obligation is in foro interno, is a breach.

The laws of nature are immutable and eternal; for injustice, ingratitude, arrogance, pride, iniquity, acception of persons, and the rest can never be made lawful. For it can never be that war shall preserve life, and peace destroy it.

The same laws, because they oblige only to a desire and endeavour, mean an unfeigned and constant endeavour, are easy to be observed. For in that they require nothing but endeavour, he that endeavoureth their performance fulfilleth them; and he that fulfilleth the law is just.

And the science of them is the true and only moral philosophy. For moral philosophy is nothing else but the science of what is good and evil in the conversation and society of mankind. Good and evil are names that signify our appetites and aversions, which in different tempers, customs, and doctrines of men are different: and diverse men differ not only in their judgement on the senses of what is pleasant and unpleasant to the taste, smell, hearing, touch, and sight; but also of what is conformable or disagreeable to reason in the actions of common life. Nay, the same man, in diverse times, differs from himself; and one time praiseth, that is, calleth good, what another time he dispraiseth, and calleth evil: from whence arise disputes, controversies, and at last war. And therefore so long as a man is in the condition of mere nature, which is a condition of war, private appetite is the measure of good and evil: and consequently all men agree on this, that peace is good, and therefore also the way or means of peace, which (as I have shown before) are justice, gratitude, modesty, equity, mercy, and the rest of the laws of nature, are good; that is to say, moral virtues; and their contrary vices, evil. Now the science of virtue and vice is moral philosophy; and therefore the true doctrine of the laws of nature is the true moral philosophy. But the writers of moral philosophy, though they acknowledge the same virtues and vices; yet, not seeing wherein consisted their goodness, nor that they come to be praised as the means of peaceable, sociable, and comfortable living, place them in a mediocrity of passions: as if not the cause, but the degree of daring, made fortitude; or not the cause, but the quantity of a gift, made liberality.

These dictates of reason men used to call by the name of laws, but improperly: for they are but conclusions or theorems concerning what conduceth to the conservation and defence of themselves; whereas law, properly, is the word of him that by right hath command over others. But yet if we consider the same theorems as delivered in the word of God that by right commandeth all things, then are they properly called laws.

Section II

Favorite American Poets

2.a. Robert Frost

Robert Frost was born in San Francisco in 1874, but moved to New England at the age of eleven in Lawrence, Massachusetts. He attended Dartmouth College in 1892, and later Harvard, but never earned a degree. Frost drifted through many occupations after leaving school, working as a teacher, cobbler, and editor of the Lawrence Sentinel. *His first professional poem, "My Butterfly," was published on November 8, 1894, in the New York newspaper* The Independent.

In 1895, Frost married Elinor Miriam White; the couple moved to England in 1912, after their New Hampshire farm failed; it was abroad that Frost met and was influenced by such contemporary British poets as Edward Thomas, Rupert Brooke, *and* Robert Graves. *While in England, Frost also established a friendship with the poet* Ezra Pound, *who helped to promote and publish his work. When Frost returned to the United States in 1915, he had published two full-length collections,* A Boy's Will *and* North of Boston, *and his reputation was established. By the nineteen-twenties, he was the most celebrated poet in America, and with each new book—including* New Hampshire *(1923),* A Further Range *(1936),* Steeple Bush *(1947), and* In the Clearing *(1962)—his fame and honors (including four Pulitzer Prizes) increased.*

Though his work is principally associated with the life and landscape of New England, Frost is anything but a regional or minor poet. The author of meditations on universal themes, he is modern by adhering to language as it is spoken. Robert Frost lived and taught for many years in Massachusetts and Vermont, and died on January 29, 1963, in Boston.

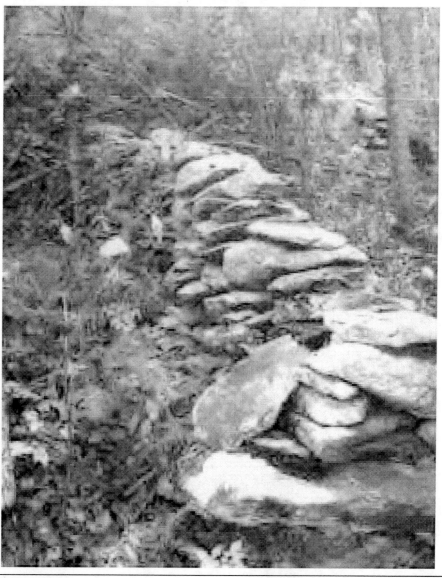

Writing about Robert Frost

Robert Frost profoundly influenced my poetry as a young girl growing up in wooded Massachusetts. In the first two poems, in true Wordsworthian manner, Frost takes an ordinary experience and transforms it into philosophical questioning of human experience. As you read the following poems, think about how real life experiences connect to Apple-picking:

- Can life be lived fully without regrets?

- Does the poem suggest something more than realistic description of an experience?

- Any symbolism in Frost's choice of words?

- Is there any type of religious meaning in this poem?

- Is the poem about picking apples or NOT picking apples?"

After Apple-Picking

My long two-pointed ladder's sticking through a tree
Toward heaven still,
And there's a barrel that I didn't fill
Beside it, and there may be two or three
Apples I didn't pick upon some bough.
But I am done with apple-picking now.
Essence of winter sleep is on the night,
The scent of apples: I am drowsing off.
I cannot rub the strangeness from my sight
I got from looking through a pane of glass
I skimmed this morning from the drinking trough
And held against the world of hoary grass.
It melted, and I let it fall and break.
But I was well
Upon my way to sleep before it fell,
And I could tell
What form my dreaming was about to take.
Magnified apples appear and disappear,
Stem end and blossom end,
And every fleck of russet showing clear.
My instep arch not only keeps the ache,
It keeps the pressure of a ladder-round.
I feel the ladder sway as the boughs bend.
And I keep hearing from the cellar bin
The rumbling sound

Of load on load of apples coming in.
For I have had too much
Of apple-picking: I am overtired
Of the great harvest I myself desired.
There were ten thousand thousand fruit to touch,
Cherish in hand, lift down, and not let fall.
For all
That struck the earth,
No matter if not bruised or spiked with stubble,
Went surely to the cider-apple heap
As of no worth.

One can see what will trouble
This sleep of mine, whatever sleep it is.
Were he not gone,
The woodchuck could say whether it's like his
Long sleep, as I describe its coming on,
Or just some human sleep.

Writing Memories and Meaning

When I studied acting at the Abbey Theatre on Dublin, Ireland, I used the following poem as an audition piece. I had earlier performed many of Frost's poems in Dublin theaters in 1976, and in an arts festival in County Limerick where I met the owner of Castle Matrix, retired Colonel U.S. Air Force and now deceased, Sean O'Driscoll. I also associate the following poem with growing up in the woods of Massachusetts when I climbed tall pines and birches, and studied baby birds in their nests. Try to listen to the speaker of the poem:

- What kind of memories is the speaker recalling?

- Can you relate to any of her memories?

- Have you ever been a swinger of birches?

- Are there levels of meaning in the poem, or is there just one meaning?

- When you think of birches, what do you see?

Birches

When I see birches bend to left and right
Across the lines of straighter darker trees,
I like to think some boy's been swinging them.
But swinging doesn't bend them down to stay.

Ice-storms do that. Often you must have seen them
Loaded with ice a sunny winter morning
After a rain. They click upon themselves
As the breeze rises, and turn many-colored
As the stir cracks and crazes their enamel.
Soon the sun's warmth makes them shed crystal shells
Shattering and avalanching on the snow-crust —
Such heaps of broken glass to sweep away
You'd think the inner dome of heaven had fallen.
They are dragged to the withered bracken by the load
And they seem not to break; though once they are bowed
So low for long they never right themselves:
You may see their trunks arching in the woods
Years afterwards, trailing their leaves on the ground
Like girls on hands and knees that throw their hair
Before them over their heads to dry in the sun.
But I was going to say when truth broke in
With all her matter-of-fact about the ice storm,
(Now am I free to be poetical?)
I should prefer to have some boy bend them
As he went out and in to fetch the cows —
Some boy too far from town to learn baseball,
Whose only play was what he found himself,
Summer or winter, and could play alone.
One by one he subdued his father's trees
By riding them down over and over again
Until he took the stiffness out of them
And not one but hung limp, not one was left
For him to conquer. He learned all there was
To learn about not launching out too soon
And so not carrying the tree away
Clear to the ground. He always kept his poise
To the top branches, climbing carefully
With the same pains you use to fill a cup
Up to the brim, and even above the brim.
Then he flung outward, feet first, with a swish,
Kicking his way down through the air to the ground.
So was I once myself a swinger of birches.
And so I dream of going back to be.
It's when I'm weary of considerations,
And life is too much like a pathless wood
Where your face burns and tickles with the cobwebs
Broken across it, and one eye is weeping

From a twig's having lashed across it open.
I'd like to get away from earth awhile
And then come back to it and begin over.
May no fate willfully misunderstand me
And half grant what I wish and snatch me away
Not to return. Earth's the right place for love:
I don't know where it's likely to go better.
I'd like to go by climbing a birch tree,
And climb black branches up a snow-white trunk
Toward heaven, till the tree could bear no more,
But dipped its top and set me down again.
That would be good both going and coming back.
One could do worse than be a swinger of birches.

Writing Life Choices

The following poem speaks of choices we face in life, and Frost believes in venturing down the less traveled road. I often have used this poem to validate choices I have made in life.

- How do you validate your choices?

- Are you conservative, moderate, liberal? Does this affect your choices?

- How would your political and religious affiliations affect your choices?

- Have you ever been faced with two choices? How did you choose?

The Road not Taken

Two roads diverged in a yellow wood,
And sorry I could not travel both
And be one traveler, long I stood
And looked down one as far as I could
To where it bent in the undergrowth;
Then took the other, as just as fair,
And having perhaps the better claim
Because it was grassy and wanted wear,
Though as for that the passing there
Had worn them really about the same,
And both that morning equally lay
In leaves no step had trodden black.
Oh, I marked the first for another day!
Yet knowing how way leads on to way

I doubted if I should ever come back.
I shall be telling this with a sigh
Somewhere ages and ages hence:
Two roads diverged in a wood, and I,
I took the one less traveled by,
And that has made all the difference.

Writing Images and Eras

2. b Allen Ginsberg

Irwin Allen Ginsberg (1926 – 1997) was an <u>American</u> <u>Beat poet</u> born in <u>Newark,</u> <u>New Jersey</u>. Ginsberg is best known for <u>Howl</u> (1956), a long poem about <u>consumer</u> <u>society</u>'s negative <u>human values</u>. Later in his life, Ginsberg formed a bridge between the <u>Beat</u> movement of the 1950s and the <u>hippies</u> of the 1960s, befriending <u>Timothy Leary</u>, <u>Gregory Corso</u>, <u>Rod McKuen</u>, and <u>Bob Dylan</u>.

I had the fortunate experience to hear Allen Ginsberg read his poetry at SUNY Buffalo shortly before his death. Although I never agreed with Ginsberg's politics, I always enjoyed the following passage from Howl *for its use of sounds and rhythms and visual language.*

- What kind of language choices does Ginsberg make?

- What types of images does he paint in his poetry?

- Do the poet's images still seem fresh after 60 years?

- Has this something to do with describing American modernity?

- What has happened in the past 60 years to make us more modern?

- How do you see modern life—how do computers, 24-hour news broadcasts, and cell phones make us postmodern?

From Howl

I saw the best minds of my generation destroyed by madness, starving hysterical naked,

dragging themselves through the negro streets at dawn looking for an angry fix,

angelheaded hipsters burning for the ancient heavenly connection to the starry dynamo in the machinery of night,

who poverty and tatters and hollow-eyed and high sat up smoking in the supernatural darkness of cold-water fiats 'doating across the tops of cities contemplating jazz,

who bared their brains to Heaven under the El and saw Mohammedan angels staggering on tenement roofs illuminated, who passed through universities with radiant cool eyes hallucinating Arkansas and Blake-light tragedy among the scholars of war,

who were expelled from the academies for crazy & publishing obscene odes on the windows of the skull,

who cowered in unshaven rooms in underwear, burning their money in wastebaskets and listening to the Terror through the wall,

who got busted in their pubic beards returning through Laredo with a belt of marijuana for New York,

who ate fire in paint hotels or drank turpentine in Paradise Alley, death, or purgatoried their torsos night after night,

with dreams, with drugs, with waking nightmares, alcohol and cock and endless balls,

incomparable blind streets of shuddering cloud and lightning in the mind leaping toward poles of Canada & Paterson, illuminating all the motionless world of Time between,

Peyote solidities of halls, backyard green tree cemetery dawns, wine drunkenness over the rooftops, storefront boroughs of teahead joyride neon blinking traffic light, sun and moon and tree vibrations in the roaring winter dusks of Brooklyn, ashcan rantings and kind king light of mind,

who chained themselves to subways for the endless ride from Battery to holy Bronx on benzedrine until the noise of wheels and children brought them down shuddering mouth-wracked and battered bleak of brain all drained of brilliance in the drear light of Zoo,

who sank all night in submarine light of Bickford's floated out and sat through the stale beer afternoon in desolate Fugazzi's, I listening to the crack of doom on the hydrogen jukebox,

who talked continuously seventy hours from park to pad to bar to Bellevue to museum to the Brooklyn Bridge,

a lost battalion of platonic conversationalists jumping down the stoops off fire escapes off windowsills off Empire State out of the moon,

yacketayakking screaming vomiting whispering facts and memories and anecdotes and eyeball kicks and shocks of hospitals and jails and wars,

whole intellects disgorged in total recall for seven days and nights with brilliant eyes, meat for the Synagogue cast on the pavement, who vanished into nowhere Zen New Jersey leaving a trail of ambiguous picture postcards of Atlantic City Hall,

suffering Eastern sweats and Tangerian bone-grindings and migraines of China under junk-withdrawal in Newark's bleak furnished room,

who wandered around and around at midnight in the railroad yard wondering where to go, and went, leaving no broken hearts,

who lit cigarettes in boxcars boxcars boxcars racketing through snow toward lonesome farms in grandfather night,

who studied Plotinus Poe St. John of the Cross telepathy and bop kaballa because the cosmos instinctively vibrated at their feet in Kansas,

who loned it through the streets of Idaho seeking visionary indian angels,

who were visionary indian angels,

who thought they were only mad when Baltimore gleamed in supernatural ecstasy,

who jumped in limousines with the Chinaman of Oklahoma on the impulse of winter midnight streetlight smalltown rain,

who lounged hungry and lonesome through Houston seeking jazz or sex or soup, and followed the brilliant Spaniard to converse about America and

Eternity, a hopeless task, and so took ship to Africa,

who disappeared into the volcanoes of Mexico leaving behind nothing but the shadow of dungarees and the lava and ash of poetry scattered in fireplace Chicago,

who reappeared on the West Coast investigating the E.B.I. in beards and shorts with big pacifist eyes sexy in their dark skin passing out incomprehensible leaflets,

who burned cigarette holes in their arms protesting the narcotic tobacco haze of Capitalism,

who distributed Supercommunist pamphlets in Union Square weeping and undressing while the sirens of Los Alamos wailed them down, and wailed down Wall, and the Staten Island ferry also wailed,

who broke down crying in white gymnasiums naked and trembling before the machinery of other skeletons,

who bit detectives in the neck and shrieked with delight in policecars for committing no crime but their own wild cooking pederasty and intoxication, who howled on their knees in the subway and were dragged off the roof waving genitals and manuscripts,

who let themselves be fucked in the ass by saintly motorcyclists, and screamed with joy,

who blew and were blown by those human seraphim, the sailors, caresses of Atlantic and Caribbean love,

who balled in the morning in the evenings in rosegardens and the grass of public parks and cemeteries scattering their semen freely to whomever come who may,

who hiccupped endlessly trying to giggle but wound up with a sob behind a partition in a Turkish Bath when the blonde & naked angel came to pierce them with a sword,

who lost their loveboys to the three old shrews of fate the one eyed shrew of the heterosexual dollar the one eyed shrew that winks out of the womb and the one eyed shrew that does nothing but sit on her ass and snip the intellectual golden threads of the craftsman's loom,

* * *

who went out whoring through Colorado in myriad stolen night-cars, N.C.,

secret hero of these poems, cocksman and Adonis of Denver—joy to the

memory of his innumerable lays of girls in empty lots & diner backyards,

moviehouses rickety rows, on mountaintops in caves or with gaunt

waitresses in familiar roadside lonely petticoat upliftings & especially secret

gas-station solipsisms of johns, & hometown alleys too

who faded out in vast sordid movies, were shifted in dreams, woke on a sudden Manhattan, and picked themselves up out of basements hungover with heartless Tokay and horrors of Third Avenue iron dreams & stumbled to unemployment offices,

who walked all night with their shoes full of blood on the snowbank docks

waiting for a door in the East River to open to a room full of steamheat and opium,

who created great suicidal dramas on the apartment cliff-banks of the Hudson under the wartime blue floodlight of the moon & their heads shall be crowned with laurel in oblivion, who ate the lamb stew of the imagination or digested the crab at the muddy bottom of the rivers of Bowery,

who wept at the romance of the streets with their pushcarts full of onions and bad music,

who sat in boxes breathing in the darkness under the bridge, and rose up to build harpsichords in their lofts,

who coughed on the sixth floor of Harlem crowned with flame under the tubercular sky surrounded by orange crates of theology,

who scribbled all night rocking and rolling over lofty incantations which in the yellow morning were stanzas of gibberish,

who cooked rotten animals lung heart feet tail borsht & tortillas dreaming of the pure vegetable kingdom,

who plunged themselves under meat trucks looking for an egg,

who threw their watches off the roof to cast their ballot for Eternity outside of Time, & alarm clocks fell on their heads every day for the next decade,

who cut their wrists three times successively unsuccessfully, gave up and were forced to open antique stores where they thought they were growing old and cried,

who were burned alive in their innocent flannel suits on Madison Avenue amid blasts of leaden verse & the tanked-up clatter of the iron regiments of fashion & the nitroglycerine shrieks of the fairies of advertising & the mustard gas of sinister intelligent editors, or were run down by the drunken taxicabs of Absolute Reality,

who jumped off the Brooklyn Bridge this actually happened and walked away unknown and forgotten into the ghostly daze of Chinatown soup alleyways & firetrucks, not even one free beer,

who sang out of their windows in despair, fell out of the subway window, jumped in the filthy Passaic, leaped on negroes, cried all over the street, danced on broken wineglasses barefoot smashed phonograph records of nostalgic European 1930'S German jazz finished the whiskey and threw up groaning into the bloody toilet, moans in their ears and the blast of colossal steam-whistles,

who barreled down the highways of the past journeying to each other's hotrod-Golgotha jail-solitude watch or Birmingham jazz incarnation,

who drove crosscountry seventytwo hours to find out if I had a vision or you had a vision or he had a vision to find out Eternity.

who journeyed to Denver, who died in Denver, who came back to Denver & waited in vain, who watched over Denver & brooded & loned in Denver and finally went away to find out the Time, & now Denver is lonesome for her heroes,

who fell on their knees in hopeless cathedrals praying for each other's salvation and light and breasts, until the soul illuminated its hair for a second,

who crashed through their minds in jail waiting for impossible criminals with golden heads and the charm of reality in their hearts who sang sweet blues to Alcatraz,

who retired to Mexico to cultivate a habit, or Rocky Mount to tender Buddhas or Tangiers to boys or Southern Pacific to the black locomotive' or Harvard to Narcissus to Woodlawn to the daisy-chain or grave,

who demanded sanity trials accusing the radio of hypnotism & were left with their insanity & their hands & a hung jury,

who threw potato salad at CCNY lecturers on Dadaism and subsequently presented themselves on the granite steps of the madhouse with shaven heads and harlequin speech of suicide, demanding instantaneous lobotomy,

and who were given instead the concrete void of insulin metrasol electricity hydrotherapy psychotherapy occupational therapy pingpong & amnesia,

who in humorless protest overturned only one symbolic pingpong table, resting briefly in catatonia,

returning years later truly bald except for a wig of blood, and tears and fingers, to the visible madman doom of the wards of the madtowns of the East,

Pilgrim State's Rockland's and Greystone's foetid halls, bickering with the echoes of the soul, rocking and rolling in the midnight solitude-bench dolmen-realms of love, dream of life a nightmare, bodies turned to stone as heavy as the moon,

with mother finally * * * * * *, and the last fantastic book flung out of the tenement window, and the last door closed at 4 AM and the last telephone slammed at the wall in reply and the last furnished room emptied down to the last piece of mental furniture, a yellow paper rose twisted on a wire hanger in the closet, and even that imaginary, nothing but a hopeful little bit of hallucination—

ah, Carl, while you are not safe I am not safe, and now you're really in the total animal soup of time—

and who therefore ran through the icy streets obsessed with a sudden flash of the alchemy of the use of the ellipse the catalog the meter & the vibrating plane, who dreamt and made incarnate gaps in Time & Space through images juxtaposed, and trapped the archangel of the soul between 2 visual images and joined the elemental verbs and set the noun and dash of consciousness together jumping with sensation of Pater Omnipotens Aeterna Deus

to recreate the syntax and measure of poor human prose and stand before you speechless and intelligent and shaking with shame, rejected yet confessing out the soul to conform to the rhythm of thought in his naked and endless head,

the madman bum and angel beat in Time, unknown, yet putting down here what might be left to say in time come after death,

and rose reincarnate in the ghostly clothes of jazz in the goldhorn shadow of the band and blew the suffering of America's naked mind for love into an eli

eli lamma lamma sabacthani saxophone cry that shivered the cities down to the last radio

with the absolute heart of the poem of life butchered out of their own bodies good to eat a thousand years.

Section III

Favorite Irish and English Poets

3.a. William Butler Yeats

William Butler Yeats (<u>1865</u> - <u>1939</u>) was an <u>Irish poet</u>, <u>dramatist</u>, <u>mystic</u> and <u>public figure</u>, brother of the artist <u>Jack Butler Yeats</u> and son of <u>John Butler Yeats</u>. Yeats was one of the driving forces behind the <u>Irish Literary Revival</u> and was co-founder of the <u>Abbey Theatre</u>. Yeats also served as an Irish <u>Senator</u>. He was awarded the <u>Nobel Prize for literature</u> in 1923.

Writing Symbols: Connecting Places and Events

When I lived in Ireland I visited Yeat's grave under Ben Bulben, and there were three white roses growing on one stem and I picked that rose. There is a small stone chapel there, and I played the pipe organ for my Irish friends. I remember my visit to Donegal, and how wild the storm and winds. I remember the swans over Kilary Harbor. I remember symbols for the places I have visited, and use these symbols to remember how my life has passed and what has driven me.

- How do you remember places and events in your own life?
- How do cultures associate with symbols?
- What symbol do we as Americans adhere to? The dollar sign? The flag? The eagle?
- How does Yeats describe his vision of Eden?
- Why did Yeats live in a tower? What is a tower a symbol of?
- Can you relate to his spiraling vision?

The Lake Isle of Innisfree

I will arise and go now, and go to Innisfree,
And a small cabin build there, of clay and wattles made:
Nine bean-rows will I have there, a hive for the honey-bee,
And live alone in the bee-loud glade.

And I shall have some peace there, for peace comes dropping slow,
Dropping from the veils of the morning to where the cricket sings;
There midnight's all a glimmer, and noon a purple glow,
And evening full of the linnet's wings.

I will arise and go now, for always night and day
I hear lake water lapping with low sounds by the shore;
While I stand on the roadway, or on the pavements grey,
I hear it in the deep heart's core.

Writing the Future: Forecasting

In "The Second Coming," Yeats tries to forecast his vision into the future—what does he see? He sees a place and time when "The best lack all conviction, while the worst Are full of passionate intensity." Is he describing a dispassionate and bored society in the future, where the dregs of society make the most noise?

- What is the poet seeing in the future?
- Do you agree or disagree that the vision was accurate?
- What is the "gyre" a symbol of?
- Who or what is the "rough beast" slouching toward Bethlehem? What do you visualize when you read the image? That of an Egyptian Sphinx?

The Second Coming

Turning and turning in the widening gyre
The falcon cannot hear the falconer;
Things fall apart; the centre cannot hold;
Mere anarchy is loosed upon the world,
The blood-dimmed tide is loosed, and everywhere
The ceremony of innocence is drowned;
The best lack all conviction, while the worst
Are full of passionate intensity.

Surely some revelation is at hand;
Surely the Second Coming is at hand.
The Second Coming! Hardly are those words out
When a vast image out of *Spiritus Mundi*
Troubles my sight: somewhere in sands of the desert
A shape with lion body and the head of a man,
A gaze blank and pitiless as the sun,
Is moving its slow thighs, while all about it
Reel shadows of the indignant desert birds.
The darkness drops again; but now I know
That twenty centuries of stony sleep
Were vexed to nightmare by a rocking cradle,
And what rough beast, its hour come round at last,
Slouches towards Bethlehem to be born?

Writing on Themes

The next poem contains sensual language sounds and should be sung. Here the poet travels in his imagination and memory to the city of Byzantium where he wants to forecast for the populace. After reading the poem think about the themes Yeats writes about:

- How does this poem relate to "The Second Coming"?

- Has Yeats developed a "theme" in his poetry?

- Do you think Yeats is a religious or philosophical writer?

- Do you often think of wanting to say something to people, but did not have the courage?

Sailing to Byzantium

I

That is no country for old men. The young
In one another's arms, birds in the trees
— Those dying generations — at their song,
The salmon-falls, the mackerel-crowded seas,
Fish, flesh, or fowl, commend all summer long
Whatever is begotten, born, and dies.
Caught in that sensual music all neglect
Monuments of unageing intellect.

II

An aged man is but a paltry thing,
A tattered coat upon a stick, unless
Soul clap its hands and sing, and louder sing
For every tatter in its mortal dress,
Nor is there singing school but studying
Monuments of its own magnificence;
And therefore I have sailed the seas and come
To the holy city of Byzantium.

III

O sages standing in God's holy fire
As in the gold mosaic of a wall
Come from the holy fire, perne in a gyre,
And be the singing-masters of my soul.
Consume my heart away; sick with desire
And fastened to a dying animal
It knows not what it is; and gather me
Into the artifice of eternity.

IV

Once out of nature I shalll never take
My bodily form from any natural thing,
But such a form as Grecian goldsmiths make
Of hammered gold and gold enamelling
To keep a drowsy Emperor awake;
Or set upon a golden bough to sing
To lords and ladies of Byzantium
Of what is past, or passing, or to come.

While in County Sligo at Yeats' grave, I saw the tombstone and read the inscription as contained in the following poems. Ben Bulben is a very high mountain and rather flat at the top. My Irish friends told me that ancient Irish queens were buried there, and that no one should ever climb that mountain. I remember not being disappointed at the prospect.

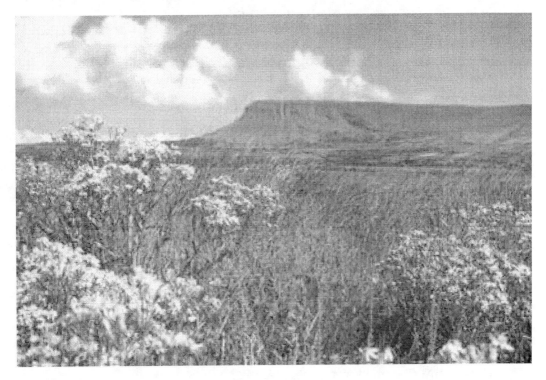

From 'Under Ben Bulben'

Under bare Ben Bulben's head
In Drumcliff churchyard Yeats is laid.
An ancestor was rector there
Long years ago, a church stands near,
By the road an ancient cross.
No marble, no conventional phrase;
On limestone quarried near the spot
By his command these words are cut:

Cast a cold eye
On life, on death.
Horseman, pass by!

3b. John Donne

John Donne (1572 –1631) was a Jacobean metaphysical poet. His works include sonnets, love poetry, religious poems, Latin translations, epigrams, elegies, songs, and sermons. I always enjoy John Donne's spirit in his eloquent verses, and I try to visualize him preaching the Gospel, as his verses are very sexy.

Writing Response

- Why does the speaker of the poem chide the sun?

- Can you relate at all to the images Donne paints of seduction, where he asks the sun to shine on his bed and make it central to the universe?

- Do you think the image is shocking? Or kind of funny because the poem is so old?

- What language speaks of sensuality in the poem?

The Sun Rising

BUSY old fool, unruly Sun,
Why dost thou thus,
Through windows, and through curtains, call on us ?
Must to thy motions lovers' seasons run ?
Saucy pedantic wretch, go chide
Late school-boys and sour prentices,
Go tell court-huntsmen that the king will ride,
Call country ants to harvest offices ;
Love, all alike, no season knows nor clime,
Nor hours, days, months, which are the rags of time.

Thy beams so reverend, and strong
Why shouldst thou think ?
I could eclipse and cloud them with a wink,
But that I would not lose her sight so long.
If her eyes have not blinded thine,
Look, and to-morrow late tell me,
Whether both th' Indias of spice and mine
Be where thou left'st them, or lie here with me.
Ask for those kings whom thou saw'st yesterday,
And thou shalt hear, "All here in one bed lay."

She's all states, and all princes I ;
Nothing else is ;
Princes do but play us ; compared to this,
All honour's mimic, all wealth alchemy.
Thou, Sun, art half as happy as we,
In that the world's contracted thus ;
Thine age asks ease, and since thy duties be
To warm the world, that's done in warming us.
Shine here to us, and thou art everywhere ;
This bed thy center is, these walls thy sphere.

Writing about Gender Relations

Donne's next poem speaks of a man complaining about his search to find a woman both "true and fair." Donne makes it seem impossible—is he sexist or just frustrated? You will find much of the language and symbols familiar.

- Do you think the media portrays woman as weak? Or portrays characteristics Donne talks about?
- Is Donne implying that a woman cannot be both beautiful and trusted?
- What is the importance of the "mandrake root"?
- Why do you think Donne wrote this poem?

Song

GO and catch a falling star,
Get with child a mandrake root,
Tell me where all past years are,
Or who cleft the devil's foot,
Teach me to hear mermaids singing,
Or to keep off envy's stinging,
And find
What wind
Serves to advance an honest mind.

If thou be'st born to strange sights,
Things invisible to see,
Ride ten thousand days and nights,
Till age snow white hairs on thee,
Thou, when thou return'st, wilt tell me,
All strange wonders that befell thee,
And swear,
No where
Lives a woman true and fair.

If thou find'st one, let me know,
Such a pilgrimage were sweet;
Yet do not, I would not go,
Though at next door we might meet,
Though she were true, when you met her,
And last, till you write your letter,
Yet she
Will be
False, ere I come, to two, or three.

Writing about the Religious

John Donne was famous for his religious meditations, and this one is my particular favorite. I don't see Donne exclusively hearing a "bell" of death ringing, but I hear him celebrating the sanctity of human life and confessing that God is our only security. I wanted the reader to experience reading the language and spelling of another time and place.

- Why has Donne made the "bell" his central image?

- What does Donne think of the human condition?

- Do you feel important in your environment?

- Do you connect to some higher power?

Meditation XVII:

From Devotions Upon Emergent Occasions

Nunc lento sonitu dicunt, Morieris

Now, this Bell tolling softly for another, saies to me, Thou must die.

PERCHANCE hee for whom this *Bell* tolls, may be so ill, as that he knowes not it tolls for him; And perchance I may thinke my selfe so much better than I am, as that they who are about mee, and see my state, may have caused it to toll for mee, and I know not that. The *Church* is *Catholike, universall,* so are all her *Actions; All* that she does, belongs to *all.* When she *baptizes a child,* that action concernes mee; for that child is thereby connected to that *Head* which is my *Head* too, and engraffed into that *body,* whereof I am a *member.* And when she *buries a Man,* that action concernes me: All *mankinde* is of one *Author,* and is one *volume;* when one Man dies, one *Chapter* is not *torne* out of the *booke,* but *translated* into a better *language;* and every *Chapter* must be so *translated; God* emploies several *translators;* some peeces are translated by *age,* some by *sicknesse,* some by warre, some by *justice;* but *Gods* hand is in every *translation;* and his hand shall binde up all our scattered leaves againe, for that *Librarie* where every *booke* shall lie open to one another: As therefore the *Bell* that rings to a *Sermon,* calls not upon the *Preacher* onely, but upon the *Congregation* to come; so this *Bell* calls us all: but how much more mee, who am brought so neere the *doore* by this sicknesse. There was a *contention* as farre as a *suite,* (in which both *pietie* and *dignitie, religion,* and *estimation,* were mingled) which of the religious *Orders* should ring to *praiers* first in the *Morning;* and it was that *they should ring first that rose earliest.* If we understand aright the *dignitie* of this *Belle* that tolls for our *evening prayer,* wee would bee glad to make it ours, by rising early, in that *application,* that it might bee ours, as wel as his, whose indeed it is. The *Bell* doth toll for him that *thinkes* it doth; and though it *intermit* againe, yet from that *minute,* that that occasion wrought upon him, hee is united to *God.* Who casts not up his *Eye* to the *Sunne* when it rises? but who takes off his *Eye* from a *Comet* when that breakes out? Who bends not his *eare* to any *bell,* which upon any occasion rings? but who can remove it from that *bell,* which is passing a *peece of himselfe* out of this *world?* No man is an *Iland,* intire of it selfe; every man is a peece of the *Continent,* a part of the *maine;* if a Clod bee washed away by the *Sea, Europe* is the lesse, as well as if a *Promontorie* were, as well as if a *Mannor* of thy *friends* or of *thine owne* were; any mans *death* diminishes *me,* because I am involved in *Mankinde;* And therefore never send to know for whom the *bell* tolls; It tolls for *thee.* Neither can we call this a *begging of Miserie* or a *borrowing of Miserie,* as though we were not miserable enough of our selves, but must fetch in more from the next house, in taking upon us the *Miserie* of our *Neighbours.* Truly it were an excusable *covetousnesse* if wee did; for *affliction* is a *treasure,* and scarce any man hath *enough* of it. No man hath *affliction* enough that is not matured, and ripened by it, and made fit for God by that *affliction.* If a man carry *treasure* in *bullion,* or in a *wedge* of *gold,* and have none coined into *currant Monies,* his *treasure* will not defray him as he travells. *Tribulation* is *Treasure* in the *nature* of it, but it is not *currant money* in the *use* of it, except wee get nearer and nearer our *home, Heaven,* by it. Another man may be sicke too, and sick to *death,* and this *affliction* may lie in his *bowels,* as *gold* in a *Mine,* and be of no use to him; but this *bell,* that tells me of his *affliction,* digs out, and applies that *gold* to *mee:* if by this consideration of anothers danger, I take mine owne into contemplation, and so secure my selfe, by making my recourse to my *God,* who is our onely securitie. (1624).

3.c. William Wordsworth

William Wordsworth (1770 - 1850) was a major English romantic poet who, with Samuel Taylor Coleridge, helped launch the Romantic movement in English literature with their 1798, Lyrical Ballads. Wordsworth's masterpiece is generally considered to be The Prelude, an autobiographical poem of his early years that was revised and expanded a number of times. It was never published during his lifetime, and was only given the title after his death (up until this time it was generally known as the poem "to Coleridge"). Wordsworth was England's Poet Laureate from 1843 until his death in 1850.

Wordsworth's Prelude opens with a literal journey whose goal is the Vale of Grasmere. The Prelude narrates a number of later journeys, most notably the crossing of the Alps in book VI and, in the beginning of the final book, the climatic ascent of Snowdon. In the course of the poem, literal journeys become the metaphorical vehicle for spiritual journeys — the journey in the poet's memory.[1]

Commentary on *the Prelude*

The following is an essay I wrote in the mid-1990s on *The Prelude*; I was invited to read the essay at Dove Cottage by Jonathan Wordsworth during the annual Wordsworth conference, but I could not fly to England that year. This essay is then followed by the famous Alps journey in Book VI of *The Prelude*.

Divinity in Imagination

" For him the poet, using no bible but nature, was the *Seer* whose keener senses and fresher and more integral imagination make him the supreme teacher, whose office it is to render men better and happier by revealing to them their own nature and that of the universe in which they dwell." (Emile Legouis 42)

Wordsworth's poetry celebrates the mysteries of man's place in the world and the wonder of the universe; however, it does not exalt mysteries that conventional religious faith considers suitable to explain human creation. Wordsworth's poetry does not demand that the reader be educated in Christian doctrines, for his poetry eschews dogma, and is not Christ-centered but imagination and creation-centered, thus making his poetry accessible to people of all sectarian beliefs.

The topical scope of possible religious implications in Wordsworth's poetry could include: Wordsworth as a religious teacher and healer of humanity through

---

1   From The Norton Anthology of English Literature, Eighth Edition 2006

nature; the poet as minister; the poet discovering his chosen status; the moral effects of communion with nature on the human mind; the recognition that a person's relationship with nature could reinforce a connection to the Deity; or, the evolution of the human soul through sensory perceptions of nature. Clearly, a detailed engagement of this range of subjects is beyond the confines of a brief encounter with the bard's religious philosophy.

Wordsworth's conviction is that intense communion with nature molds the human consciousness, creating the potential for access to new spiritual dimensions within the human soul, mind, and imagination. Thus, a focus on the religious symbolism of nature images, such as water and light, and a concentration on the elevation of the human imagination to divine proportions, through heightened sense perceptions provoked by nature, which invoke apocalyptic visions, in selected passages from *The Prelude*, may provide an entrance to spiritual dimensions of Wordsworth's poetry.

Throughout *The Prelude*, Wordsworth traces the growth of imagination in the creative mind of the poet. Wordsworth's meditations of nature combine concepts of mind and perception, that is, imagination and sensory input, as functions which elevate imagination to divinely creative proportions, a relationship that connects the human soul to the spiritual world of that which is both seen and unseen. Stephen Gill writes about this subject that, "Wordsworth...presents the mind in perception as vitally active, engaged in a constant act of creation-in-perception. Truly creative minds, Wordsworth asserts, both are from the Deity and partake of the nature of the Deity" (Gill 91). A brief example follows of the poet traversing the chasm between the human mind and divine power, a chasm which becomes bridged when imagination, through the inspiration of acute sensory perceptions, enables the mind to become empowered with god-like creative dimensions:

> "...- yet I have stood
> even while mine eye has moved o'er three long leagues
> of shining water, gathering, as it seemed,
> Through every hair-breadth of that field of light
> New pleasure..." (I.604-608)

Wordsworth evokes the creation in the transcendent quality of his experience, by turning shining water into a field of light. According to the book of Genesis, God's first act of creation was that of dissolving the darkness that was upon "...the face of the deep" into light (Genesis I.2). God's second act, according to the same chapter, was the creation of waters. In both acts of creation, "God saw that it was good." In the above poetic passage, the poet becomes a divine creator, dissolving water into light, as his "eye" becomes the creative center of his imaginative power, "gathering... pleasure" for the poet, a satisfaction reportedly shared by the Divine Creator in the Genesis account. That the human senses are capable of transforming and transposing nature's immutable forms through mind and imagination, and are able to recreate new forms, natural forms generally considered unchangeable, through human creative powers, indicates that Wordsworth connects the potential of the human mind and imagination to divine dimensions - limitless and unrestricted. As Jonathan Wordsworth has written, "With the primary imagination man unknowingly reenacts God's original and eternal creative moment" (Wordsworth 25).

The thematic concern of Book VI, lines 525-572, centers on imagination as a topic for meditation, and as being the prime source of power which equips the mind to experience visions of the "...characters of the great apocalypse." Wordsworth praises and recognizes the "glory of my soul," after a religious vision of his imagination transcending like some divinely mystical "unfathered vapour." His visions, "...visitings of awful promise," lift the poet to a spiritual dimension which ordinarily can neither be experienced nor seen, that aspect of the spiritual realm which can only be sense-penetrated by the "light of sense" going "out in flashes," by a higher perception of spiritual enlightenment. The poet understands that this normally unseen spiritual realm is where "greatness makes abode," the final, eternal habitation for the divine essence in humans - imagination.

What Wordsworth had hoped to experience in crossing the Alps in full consciousness had slipped by, unnoticed, when he discovered through a chance encounter with a stranger that he had already crossed the Alps. Deep dejection overwhelmed him. Yet, what Wordsworth came for, he did not discover on the mountain peaks, but in his descent to the Ravine of Gondo.

> "...The immeasurable height
> of woods decaying, never to be decayed,
> The stationary blasts of waterfalls,
> And everywhere along the hollow rent
> Winds thwarting winds, bewildered and forlorn,
> The torrents shooting from the clear blue sky,
> The rocks that muttered close upon our ears-
> Black drizzling crags that spake by the wayside
> As if a voice were in them - the sickly sight
> And giddy prospect of the raving stream,
> The unfettered clouds and region of the heavens,
> Tumult and peace, the darkness and the light,
> Were all like workings of one mind, the features
> Of the same face, blossoms upon one tree,
> Characters of the great apocalypse,
> The types and symbols of eternity,
> Of first, and last, and midst, and without end."

Geoffrey Hartman, in commenting on Wordsworth's apocalyptic vision of the Alpine experience, states that "Nature seems to have guided the travelers to a point where they see the power which causes it to move and be moving. This power, when distinct from nature, is called Imagination" (Hartman 192).

Wordsworth discovers, finally, that true "greatness" does not involve conquering literal heights, not in the accomplishment of "spoils and trophies" which attest to man's physical prowess, but in developing receptivity to spiritual "...visitings/Of awful promise that have shown to us/The invisible world."(VI.525-29;535-36) It is the imagination and the soul's connection to this higher "promise" or power, forces amplified by heightened sense perceptions, that have imbued humans with divinity, the power to reach through the limited dimensions of the earthly plane, and to penetrate through that spiritual dimension of what normally is "unseen." To advance and illuminate Hartman's explanation - nature is the guide, the senses are the operational vehicle for viewing nature's omnipotence, and imagination is the receptive power of this grandeur, a naturally receptive, human power separate from nature and inherent in the human mind.

The image of "infinitude," the eternal habitation for the divine essence (imagination) in man, is reiterated in the image of the "immeasurable height of woods decaying, never to be decayed." Wordsworth's spiritual odyssey is compounded by the assault on his senses by the powerful elements of natures, which all speak of God: the "stationary blasts of waterfalls," "winds thwarting winds," "torrents shooting from the clear, blue sky," the personification of the muttering rocks, the images of speaking crags and "raving streams." These elemental forces, the engraved characters of God's most awesome demonstration of his power on earth, become unified forces within the poet's imagination as "one mind," "the same face," and are premonitions of the power of the "great apocalypse," the revelation of the true meaning of "infinitude." Once again, Wordsworth presents his tenet that human consciousness, through heightened sense perceptions of nature, raises the human imagination to divine proportions, allowing us to glimpse flashes of the final apocalypse, God's last revelation to mankind.

The poet's first ascent to the Alps and his second ascent to Mount Snowdon may be likened to the ancient stories of prophets ascending mountains in search of direct encounters and revelations from God. In his ascent to Mount Snowdon, Wordsworth once again describes imagination at work. His reported experience on this mountain is a rich exposition of the significance of the creative mind, provoked through sensory perceptions, which merges natural elements with a concept of the divine:

"...at my feet the ground appeared to brighten,
And with a step or two seemed brighter still;
Nor had I time to ask the cause of this,

For instantly a light upon the turf
Fell like a flash. I looked about, and lo,
the moon stood naked in the heavens at height
Immense above my head, and on the shore
I found myself of a huge sea of mist,
Which meek and silent rested at my feet.
A hundred hills their dusky backs upheaved
All over this still ocean, and beyond,
Far, far beyond, the vapours shot themselves
In headlands, tongues, and promontory shapes,

                      Into the sea, the real sea, that seemed
To dwindle and give up its majesty,
Usurped upon as far as sight could reach.
Meanwhile the moon looked down upon this shew
In single glory, and we stood, the mist
Touching our very feet; and from the shore
At distance not a third part of a mile
Was a blue chasm, a fracture in the vapour,
A deep and gloomy breathing place, through which
Mounted the roar of waters, torrents, streams
Innumerable, roaring with one voice.
The universal spectacle throughout
Was shaped for admiration and delight,
Grand in itself alone, but in that breach
Through which the homeless waters rose,
That dark, deep thoroughfare, had Nature lodged
The soul, the imagination of the whole."(XIII.35-65)

The "flash of light," which the poet speaks of, is the light signifying the presence of the divine, the light which carries revelation, a light only experienced by mystics in search of ultimate truth and enlightenment. It is not startling, then, to discover that the scriptures have already told us: "O Lord my God, Thou art very great!...Who coverest Thyself with light as with a garment." (Psalms 104:1-2) Nor are we astonished to discover that "...in Thy light do we see light."(Psalms 36:9) However, as the poet looks about for the source of the light, he sees a naked moon. Thus, the source of the light signifying revelation and divine presence is the reception of heightened sensory perceptions of a natural phenomenon, namely the moon.

In *The Confessional Imagination*, Frank Mcconnell says of this passage that "It is a vision of things at their vanishing point, returning to the primal state of indeterminacy in which all shapes and transformations are possible - yet at the same time, things revealing, in their very malleability, their eternal presence and the everlasting mystery of their substance" (Mcconnell 154). What Mcconnell fails to include in his explication of this passage is that the possibility of shapes and transformations dwell in the mind's ability, through creative transmutation, to alter the perceptions of what is seen in reality to what is seen in the imagination. In this lies the mystery of "things" transformed.

Here, on Mount Snowdon, the whole world appears under the revelation of the moonlight to be returned to its primal state of water. The mist below is the silent sea, the hills around have become static billows; and this illusory sea stretches out into the real Atlantic. Suddenly, through a "chasm" in the midst of the watery imagery, Wordsworth hears the roar of inland waters, an abrupt sensory movement from sight to sound. The poet has experienced a manifestation of the pure potentiality of imagination, for he has beheld, in the moon over the waters, the "perfect image of a mighty mind"(69) brooding over an abyss - waiting, like God, to bring forth the world. It was in this auditory, sensory experience of the chasm, that Wordsworth had experienced the abyss of the soul, the eternal habitation for man's imagination, limitless in power and creativity.

The meditation on the creative mind, immediately follows the Mount Snowdon episode:

"The perfect image of a mighty mind,
Of one that feeds upon infinity,
That is exalted by an under-presence,
The sense of God, or whatso'er is dim
Or vast in its own being...

....in a world of life they live,
By sensible impressions not enthralled,
But quickened, rouzed, and made thereby more fit
To hold communion with the invisible world.
Such minds are truly from the Deity." (69-105)

Nature translates the dialect of the soul into the language of the senses, provoking the human mind, though the imagination, to a higher state of consciousness, the very palpable perception of God's presence. The "mighty mind," has the capacity to perceive Divine presence through the energy and power of its sense perceptions of nature, processed through the divine imagination of man. The poet also recognizes that this special human ability, this imagination, is a gift from the Divine source of creation that allows the human mind to "hold communion with the invisible world."

Imagination, for Wordsworth, is the sacred power that connects human consciousness to Divine Creator consciousness, enabling the human mind to recreate the generally immutable forms of nature into forms that signify divine revelations. The capacity of human imagination must combine with a reasoned will to achieve the self-affirming act of achieving divinity in imagination. Man has not just the capacity to become angelic because, as Jonathan Wordsworth has pointed out, "...the soul is reason's being (Wordsworth 37);" man has the capacity to become a god, indeed, has been declared to have been created a god: "I say, `You are gods, sons of the Most High, all of you." (Psalms 2:6)

There is nothing conventionally religious in Wordsworth's attitudes towards God. Conventional, Christian religion espouses doctrines of Christ-centeredness, whereas Wordsworth's beliefs center on nature as creation, and human imagination as a divine creative force reacting to and upon creation, provoking the human mind to elevated states of consciousness. This philosophy shuns the idea of man as a created object, and establishes the belief that man, through the self-naming powers of his imagination, is able to merge as both subject and object with the natural, created world, becoming both God and Father, just as Christ has declared, "Both I and the Father are One." Therefore, the perception of God as an object, through the power of the creative imagination, must merge with man's self-consciousness to grasp the subjective thoughts, which make him a god, an exercise of the primary imagination. Just as Jehovah named himself to Moses as I AM, man's creative consciousness is able to affirm the existence of something beyond the human self. "I" and the great "I AM" become one. God, then, becomes the internal (rather than the external) shaping force that propels the existence of imagination, if so willed by the conscious and active reason of the human mind.

The human soul is then united to the "unseen" spiritual world through the input of sensory perceptions of nature, perceptions which are then converted, by human creative imagination, into limitless recreated forms, endowing the human potential with Divine creative possibilities, empowering the human consciousness to enter the wonders of divine revelation and apocalypse.

Works Cited

Bewell, Alan. *Wordsworth and the Enlightenment*. New Haven and London: Yale University Press, 1989.

Brantley, Richard E. *Wordsworth's "Natural Methodism."* New Haven and London: Yale University Press, 1975.

Gill, Stephen. *Wordsworth, The Prelude*. Cambridge: Cambridge University Press, 1991.

Gravil, Richard, Newlyn, Lucy, and Roe, Nicholas, eds. *Coleridge's Imagination*. Cambridge: Cambridge University Press, 1985.

Gravil, Richard and Harvey, W.J., eds. *Wordsworth:The Prelude*. London: Macmillan, 1987.

Hartm an, Geoffrey "A Poet's Progress: Wordsworth and the Via Naturaliter Negativa," *Wordsworth:The Prelude*, ed. Richard Gravil and W.J. Harvey. London: Macmillan Education Ltd., 1987.

Mcconnell, Frank D. *The Confessional Imagination*. Baltimore and London: The Johns Hopkins University Press, 1974.

Ober, Warren U. and Thomas, W.K. *A Mind For Ever Voyaging*. Edmonton: The University of Alberta Press, 1989.

Prickett, Stephen. *Romanticism and Religion*. Cambridge: Cambridge University Press, 1976.

Rylestone, Anne L. *Prophetic Memory in Wordsworth's Ecclesiastical Sonnets*. Carbondale and Edwardsville: Southern Illinois University Press, 1991.

Watson, J.R. *Wordsworth's Vital Soul*. Atlantic Highlands, New Jersey: Humanities Press, 1982.

Wordsworth, Jonathan. *The Borders of Vision*. Oxford: Clarendon Press, 1982.

Wordsworth, Jonathan. 'The Infinite I AM: Coleridge and the Ascent of Being.' From: Gravil, Richard and Lucy Newlyn, et al., eds. *Coleridge's Imagination: Essays in Memory of Pete Laver*. Cambridge: Cambridge University Press, 1985.

The Prelude

Book VI

Cambridge and the ALPS

THE leaves were fading when to Esthwaite's banks
And the simplicities of cottage life
I bade farewell; and, one among the youth
Who, summoned by that season, reunite
As scattered birds troop to the fowler's lure,
Went back to Granta's cloisters, not so prompt
Or eager, though as gay and undepressed
In mind, as when I thence had taken flight
A few short months before. I turned my face
Without repining from the coves and heights   10
Clothed in the sunshine of the withering fern;
Quitted, not loth, the mild magnificence
Of calmer lakes and louder streams; and you,
Frank-hearted maids of rocky Cumberland,
You and your not unwelcome days of mirth,

Relinquished, and your nights of revelry,
And in my own unlovely cell sate down
In lightsome mood—such privilege has youth
That cannot take long leave of pleasant thoughts.

The bonds of indolent society   20
Relaxing in their hold, henceforth I lived
More to myself. Two winters may be passed
Without a separate notice: many books
Were skimmed, devoured, or studiously perused,
But with no settled plan. I was detached
Internally from academic cares;
Yet independent study seemed a course
Of hardy disobedience toward friends
And kindred, proud rebellion and unkind.
This spurious virtue, rather let it bear   30
A name it now deserves, this cowardice,
Gave treacherous sanction to that over-love
Of freedom which encouraged me to turn
From regulations even of my own
As from restraints and bonds. Yet who can tell—
Who knows what thus may have been gained, both then
And at a later season, or preserved;
What love of nature, what original strength
Of contemplation, what intuitive truths
The deepest and the best, what keen research,   40
Unbiassed, unbewildered, and unawed?

The Poet's soul was with me at that time;
Sweet meditations, the still overflow
Of present happiness, while future years
Lacked not anticipations, tender dreams,
No few of which have since been realised;
And some remain, hopes for my future life.
Four years and thirty, told this very week,
Have I been now a sojourner on earth,
By sorrow not unsmitten; yet for me   50
Life's morning radiance hath not left the hills,
Her dew is on the flowers. Those were the days
Which also first emboldened me to trust
With firmness, hitherto but slightly touched
By such a daring thought, that I might leave
Some monument behind me which pure hearts

Should reverence. The instinctive humbleness,
Maintained even by the very name and thought
Of printed books and authorship, began
To melt away; and further, the dread awe 60
Of mighty names was softened down and seemed
Approachable, admitting fellowship
Of modest sympathy. Such aspect now,
Though not familiarly, my mind put on,
Content to observe, to achieve, and to enjoy.

All winter long, whenever free to choose,
Did I by night frequent the College grove
And tributary walks; the last, and oft
The only one, who had been lingering there
Through hours of silence, till the porter's bell, 70
A punctual follower on the stroke of nine,
Rang with its blunt unceremonious voice;
Inexorable summons! Lofty elms,
Inviting shades of opportune recess,
Bestowed composure on a neighbourhood
Unpeaceful in itself. A single tree
With sinuous trunk, boughs exquisitely wreathed,
Grew there; an ash which Winter for himself
Decked out with pride, and with outlandish grace:
Up from the ground, and almost to the top, 80
The trunk and every master branch were green
With clustering ivy, and the lightsome twigs
And outer spray profusely tipped with seeds
That hung in yellow tassels, while the air
Stirred them, not voiceless. Often have I stood
Foot-bound uplooking at this lovely tree
Beneath a frosty moon. The hemisphere
Of magic fiction, verse of mine perchance
May never tread; but scarcely Spenser's self
Could have more tranquil visions in his youth, 90
Or could more bright appearances create
Of human forms with superhuman powers,
Than I beheld, loitering on calm clear nights
Alone, beneath this fairy work of earth.

On the vague reading of a truant youth
'Twere idle to descant. My inner judgment
Not seldom differed from my taste in books,

As if it appertained to another mind,
And yet the books which then I valued most
Are dearest to me 'now'; for, having scanned, 100
Not heedlessly, the laws, and watched the forms
Of Nature, in that knowledge I possessed
A standard, often usefully applied,
Even when unconsciously, to things removed
From a familiar sympathy.—In fine,
I was a better judge of thoughts than words,
Misled in estimating words, not only
By common inexperience of youth,
But by the trade in classic niceties,
The dangerous craft, of culling term and phrase 110
From languages that want the living voice
To carry meaning to the natural heart;
To tell us what is passion, what is truth,
What reason, what simplicity and sense.

Yet may we not entirely overlook
The pleasure gathered from the rudiments
Of geometric science. Though advanced
In these enquiries, with regret I speak,
No farther than the threshold, there I found
Both elevation and composed delight: 120
With Indian awe and wonder, ignorance pleased
With its own struggles, did I meditate
On the relation those abstractions bear
To Nature's laws, and by what process led,
Those immaterial agents bowed their heads
Duly to serve the mind of earth-born man;
From star to star, from kindred sphere to sphere,
From system on to system without end.

More frequently from the same source I drew
A pleasure quiet and profound, a sense 130
Of permanent and universal sway,
And paramount belief; there, recognised
A type, for finite natures, of the one
Supreme Existence, the surpassing life
Which—to the boundaries of space and time,
Of melancholy space and doleful time,
Superior and incapable of change,
Nor touched by welterings of passion—is,

And hath the name of, God. Transcendent peace
And silence did await upon these thoughts   140
That were a frequent comfort to my youth.

'Tis told by one whom stormy waters threw,
With fellow-sufferers by the shipwreck spared,
Upon a desert coast, that having brought
To land a single volume, saved by chance,
A treatise of Geometry, he wont,
Although of food and clothing destitute,
And beyond common wretchedness depressed,
To part from company and take this book
(Then first a self-taught pupil in its truths)   150
To spots remote, and draw his diagrams
With a long staff upon the sand, and thus
Did oft beguile his sorrow, and almost
Forget his feeling: so (if like effect
From the same cause produced, 'mid outward things
So different, may rightly be compared),
So was it then with me, and so will be
With Poets ever. Mighty is the charm
Of those abstractions to a mind beset
With images and haunted by herself,   160
And specially delightful unto me
Was that clear synthesis built up aloft
So gracefully; even then when it appeared
Not more than a mere plaything, or a toy
To sense embodied: not the thing it is
In verity, an independent world,
Created out of pure intelligence.

Such dispositions then were mine unearned
By aught, I fear, of genuine desert—
Mine, through heaven's grace and inborn aptitudes.   170
And not to leave the story of that time
Imperfect, with these habits must be joined,
Moods melancholy, fits of spleen, that loved
A pensive sky, sad days, and piping winds,
The twilight more than dawn, autumn than spring;
A treasured and luxurious gloom of choice
And inclination mainly, and the mere
Redundancy of youth's contentedness.
—To time thus spent, add multitudes of hours

Pilfered away, by what the Bard who sang   180
Of the Enchanter Indolence hath called
"Good-natured lounging," and behold a map
Of my collegiate life—far less intense
Than duty called for, or, without regard
To duty, 'might' have sprung up of itself
By change of accidents, or even, to speak
Without unkindness, in another place.
Yet why take refuge in that plea?—the fault,
This I repeat, was mine; mine be the blame.

In summer, making quest for works of art,   190
Or scenes renowned for beauty, I explored
That streamlet whose blue current works its way
Between romantic Dovedale's spiry rocks;
Pried into Yorkshire dales, or hidden tracts
Of my own native region, and was blest
Between these sundry wanderings with a joy
Above all joys, that seemed another morn
Risen on mid noon; blest with the presence, Friend
Of that sole Sister, her who hath been long
Dear to thee also, thy true friend and mine,   200
Now, after separation desolate,
Restored to me—such absence that she seemed
A gift then first bestowed. The varied banks
Of Emont, hitherto unnamed in song,
And that monastic castle, 'mid tall trees,
Low standing by the margin of the stream,
A mansion visited (as fame reports)
By Sidney, where, in sight of our Helvellyn,
Or stormy Cross-fell, snatches he might pen
Of his Arcadia, by fraternal love   210
Inspired;—that river and those mouldering towers
Have seen us side by side, when, having clomb
The darksome windings of a broken stair,
And crept along a ridge of fractured wall,
Not without trembling, we in safety looked
Forth, through some Gothic window's open space,
And gathered with one mind a rich reward
From the far-stretching landscape, by the light
Of morning beautified, or purple eve;
Or, not less pleased, lay on some turret's head,   220
Catching from tufts of grass and hare-bell flowers
Their faintest whisper to the passing breeze,
Given out while mid-day heat oppressed the plains.

Another maid there was, who also shed
A gladness o'er that season, then to me,
By her exulting outside look of youth
And placid under-countenance, first endeared;
That other spirit, Coleridge! who is now
So near to us, that meek confiding heart,
So reverenced by us both. O'er paths and fields   230
In all that neighbourhood, through narrow lanes
Of eglantine, and through the shady woods,
And o'er the Border Beacon, and the waste
Of naked pools, and common crags that lay
Exposed on the bare fell, were scattered love,
The spirit of pleasure, and youth's golden gleam.
O Friend! we had not seen thee at that time,
And yet a power is on me, and a strong
Confusion, and I seem to plant thee there.
Far art thou wandered now in search of health   240
And milder breezes,—melancholy lot!
But thou art with us, with us in the past,
The present, with us in the times to come.
There is no grief, no sorrow, no despair,
No languor, no dejection, no dismay,
No absence scarcely can there be, for those
Who love as we do. Speed thee well! divide
With us thy pleasure; thy returning strength,
Receive it daily as a joy of ours;
Share with us thy fresh spirits, whether gift   250
Of gales Etesian or of tender thoughts.

I, too, have been a wanderer; but, alas!
How different the fate of different men.
Though mutually unknown, yea nursed and reared
As if in several elements, we were framed
To bend at last to the same discipline,
Predestined, if two beings ever were,
To seek the same delights, and have one health,
One happiness. Throughout this narrative,
Else sooner ended, I have borne in mind   260
For whom it registers the birth, and marks the growth,
Of gentleness, simplicity, and truth,
And joyous loves, that hallow innocent days
Of peace and self-command. Of rivers, fields,
And groves I speak to thee, my Friend! to thee,

Who, yet a liveried schoolboy, in the depths
Of the huge city, on the leaded roof
Of that wide edifice, thy school and home,
Wert used to lie and gaze upon the clouds
Moving in heaven; or, of that pleasure tired,   270
To shut thine eyes, and by internal light
See trees, and meadows, and thy native stream,
Far distant, thus beheld from year to year
Of a long exile. Nor could I forget,
In this late portion of my argument,
That scarcely, as my term of pupilage
Ceased, had I left those academic bowers
When thou wert thither guided. From the heart
Of London, and from cloisters there, thou camest.
And didst sit down in temperance and peace,   280
A rigorous student. What a stormy course
Then followed. Oh! it is a pang that calls
For utterance, to think what easy change
Of circumstances might to thee have spared
A world of pain, ripened a thousand hopes,
For ever withered. Through this retrospect
Of my collegiate life I still have had
Thy after-sojourn in the self-same place
Present before my eyes, have played with times
And accidents as children do with cards,   290
Or as a man, who, when his house is built,
A frame locked up in wood and stone, doth still,
As impotent fancy prompts, by his fireside,
Rebuild it to his liking. I have thought
Of thee, thy learning, gorgeous eloquence,
And all the strength and plumage of thy youth,
Thy subtle speculations, toils abstruse
Among the schoolmen, and Platonic forms
Of wild ideal pageantry, shaped out
From things well-matched or ill, and words for things,   300
The self-created sustenance of a mind
Debarred from Nature's living images,
Compelled to be a life unto herself,
And unrelentingly possessed by thirst
Of greatness, love, and beauty. Not alone,
Ah! surely not in singleness of heart
Should I have seen the light of evening fade
From smooth Cam's silent waters: had we met,

Even at that early time, needs must I trust
In the belief, that my maturer age,   310
My calmer habits, and more steady voice,
Would with an influence benign have soothed,
Or chased away, the airy wretchedness
That battened on thy youth. But thou hast trod
A march of glory, which doth put to shame
These vain regrets; health suffers in thee, else
Such grief for thee would be the weakest thought
That ever harboured in the breast of man.

A passing word erewhile did lightly touch
On wanderings of my own, that now embraced   320
With livelier hope a region wider far.

When the third summer freed us from restraint,
A youthful friend, he too a mountaineer,
Not slow to share my wishes, took his staff,
And sallying forth, we journeyed side by side,
Bound to the distant Alps. A hardy slight,
Did this unprecedented course imply,
Of college studies and their set rewards;
Nor had, in truth, the scheme been formed by me
Without uneasy forethought of the pain,   330
The censures, and ill-omening, of those
To whom my worldly interests were dear.
But Nature then was sovereign in my mind,
And mighty forms, seizing a youthful fancy,
Had given a charter to irregular hopes.
In any age of uneventful calm
Among the nations, surely would my heart
Have been possessed by similar desire;
But Europe at that time was thrilled with joy,
France standing on the top of golden hours,   340
And human nature seeming born again.

Lightly equipped, and but a few brief looks
Cast on the white cliffs of our native shore
From the receding vessel's deck, we chanced
To land at Calais on the very eve
Of that great federal day; and there we saw,
In a mean city, and among a few,
How bright a face is worn when joy of one

Is joy for tens of millions. Southward thence
We held our way, direct through hamlets, towns,   350
Gaudy with reliques of that festival,
Flowers left to wither on triumphal arcs,
And window-garlands. On the public roads,
And, once, three days successively, through paths
By which our toilsome journey was abridged,
Among sequestered villages we walked
And found benevolence and blessedness
Spread like a fragrance everywhere, when spring
Hath left no corner of the land untouched;
Where elms for many and many a league in files   360
With their thin umbrage, on the stately roads
Of that great kingdom, rustled o'er our heads,
For ever near us as we paced along:
How sweet at such a time, with such delight
On every side, in prime of youthful strength,
To feed a Poet's tender melancholy
And fond conceit of sadness, with the sound
Of undulations varying as might please
The wind that swayed them; once, and more than once,
Unhoused beneath the evening star we saw   370
Dances of liberty, and, in late hours
Of darkness, dances in the open air
Deftly prolonged, though grey-haired lookers on
Might waste their breath in chiding.
                                        Under hills—
The vine-clad hills and slopes of Burgundy,
Upon the bosom of the gentle Saone
We glided forward with the flowing stream.
Swift Rhone! thou wert the 'wings' on which we cut
A winding passage with majestic ease
Between thy lofty rocks. Enchanting show   380
Those woods and farms and orchards did present,
And single cottages and lurking towns,
Reach after reach, succession without end
Of deep and stately vales! A lonely pair
Of strangers, till day closed, we sailed along
Clustered together with a merry crowd
Of those emancipated, a blithe host
Of travellers, chiefly delegates, returning
From the great spousals newly solemnised
At their chief city, in the sight of Heaven.   390

Like bees they swarmed, gaudy and gay as bees;
Some vapoured in the unruliness of joy,
And with their swords flourished as if to fight
The saucy air. In this proud company
We landed—took with them our evening meal,
Guests welcome almost as the angels were
To Abraham of old. The supper done,
With flowing cups elate and happy thoughts
We rose at signal given, and formed a ring
And, hand in hand, danced round and round the board; 400
All hearts were open, every tongue was loud
With amity and glee; we bore a name
Honoured in France, the name of Englishmen,
And hospitably did they give us hail,
As their forerunners in a glorious course;
And round and round the board we danced again.
With these blithe friends our voyage we renewed
At early dawn. The monastery bells
Made a sweet jingling in our youthful ears;
The rapid river flowing without noise, 410
And each uprising or receding spire
Spake with a sense of peace, at intervals
Touching the heart amid the boisterous crew
By whom we were encompassed. Taking leave
Of this glad throng, foot-travellers side by side,
Measuring our steps in quiet, we pursued
Our journey, and ere twice the sun had set
Beheld the Convent of Chartreuse, and there
Rested within an awful 'solitude':
Yes, for even then no other than a place 420
Of soul-affecting 'solitude' appeared
That far-famed region, though our eyes had seen,
As toward the sacred mansion we advanced,
Arms flashing, and a military glare
Of riotous men commissioned to expel
The blameless inmates, and belike subvert
That frame of social being, which so long
Had bodied forth the ghostliness of things
In silence visible and perpetual calm.
—"Stay, stay your sacrilegious hands!"—The voice 430
Was Nature's, uttered from her Alpine throne;
I heard it then and seem to hear it now—
"Your impious work forbear, perish what may,

Let this one temple last, be this one spot
Of earth devoted to eternity!"
She ceased to speak, but while St. Bruno's pines
Waved their dark tops, not silent as they waved,
And while below, along their several beds,
Murmured the sister streams of Life and Death,
Thus by conflicting passions pressed, my heart   440
Responded; "Honour to the patriot's zeal!
Glory and hope to new-born Liberty!
Hail to the mighty projects of the time!
Discerning sword that Justice wields, do thou
Go forth and prosper; and, ye purging fires,
Up to the loftiest towers of Pride ascend,
Fanned by the breath of angry Providence.
But oh! if Past and Future be the wings
On whose support harmoniously conjoined
Moves the great spirit of human knowledge, spare   450
These courts of mystery, where a step advanced
Between the portals of the shadowy rocks
Leaves far behind life's treacherous vanities,
For penitential tears and trembling hopes
Exchanged—to equalise in God's pure sight
Monarch and peasant: be the house redeemed
With its unworldly votaries, for the sake
Of conquest over sense, hourly achieved
Through faith and meditative reason, resting
Upon the word of heaven-imparted truth,   460
Calmly triumphant; and for humbler claim
Of that imaginative impulse sent
From these majestic floods, yon shining cliffs,
The untransmuted shapes of many worlds,
Cerulean ether's pure inhabitants,
These forests unapproachable by death,
That shall endure as long as man endures,
To think, to hope, to worship, and to feel,
To struggle, to be lost within himself
In trepidation, from the blank abyss   470
To look with bodily eyes, and be consoled."
Not seldom since that moment have I wished
That thou, O Friend! the trouble or the calm
Hadst shared, when, from profane regards apart,
In sympathetic reverence we trod

The floors of those dim cloisters, till that hour,
From their foundation, strangers to the presence
Of unrestricted and unthinking man.
Abroad, how cheeringly the sunshine lay
Upon the open lawns! Vallombre's groves   480
Entering, we fed the soul with darkness; thence
Issued, and with uplifted eyes beheld,
In different quarters of the bending sky,
The cross of Jesus stand erect, as if
Hands of angelic powers had fixed it there,
Memorial reverenced by a thousand storms;
Yet then, from the undiscriminating sweep
And rage of one State-whirlwind, insecure.

'Tis not my present purpose to retrace
That variegated journey step by step.   490
A march it was of military speed,
And Earth did change her images and forms
Before us, fast as clouds are changed in heaven.
Day after day, up early and down late,
From hill to vale we dropped, from vale to hill
Mounted—from province on to province swept,
Keen hunters in a chase of fourteen weeks,
Eager as birds of prey, or as a ship
Upon the stretch, when winds are blowing fair:
Sweet coverts did we cross of pastoral life,   500
Enticing valleys, greeted them and left
Too soon, while yet the very flash and gleam
Of salutation were not passed away.
Oh! sorrow for the youth who could have seen,
Unchastened, unsubdued, unawed, unraised
To patriarchal dignity of mind,
And pure simplicity of wish and will,
Those sanctified abodes of peaceful man,
Pleased (though to hardship born, and compassed round
With danger, varying as the seasons change),   510
Pleased with his daily task, or, if not pleased,
Contented, from the moment that the dawn
(Ah! surely not without attendant gleams
Of soul-illumination) calls him forth
To industry, by glistenings flung on rocks,
Whose evening shadows lead him to repose.

Well might a stranger look with bounding heart
Down on a green recess, the first I saw
Of those deep haunts, an aboriginal vale,
Quiet and lorded over and possessed   520
By naked huts, wood-built, and sown like tents
Or Indian cabins over the fresh lawns
And by the river side.
                That very day,
From a bare ridge we also first beheld
Unveiled the summit of Mont Blanc, and grieved
To have a soulless image on the eye
That had usurped upon a living thought
That never more could be. The wondrous Vale
Of Chamouny stretched far below, and soon
With its dumb cataracts and streams of ice,   530
A motionless array of mighty waves,
Five rivers broad and vast, made rich amends,
And reconciled us to realities;
There small birds warble from the leafy trees,
The eagle soars high in the element,
There doth the reaper bind the yellow sheaf,
The maiden spread the haycock in the sun,
While Winter like a well-tamed lion walks,
Descending from the mountain to make sport
Among the cottages by beds of flowers.   540

Whate'er in this wide circuit we beheld,
Or heard, was fitted to our unripe state
Of intellect and heart. With such a book
Before our eyes, we could not choose but read
Lessons of genuine brotherhood, the plain
And universal reason of mankind,
The truths of young and old. Nor, side by side
Pacing, two social pilgrims, or alone
Each with his humour, could we fail to abound
In dreams and fictions, pensively composed: 550
Dejection taken up for pleasure's sake,
And gilded sympathies, the willow wreath,
And sober posies of funereal flowers,
Gathered among those solitudes sublime
From formal gardens of the lady Sorrow,
Did sweeten many a meditative hour.

Yet still in me with those soft luxuries
Mixed something of stern mood, an underthirst
Of vigour seldom utterly allayed:
And from that source how different a sadness   560
Would issue, let one incident make known.
When from the Vallais we had turned, and clomb
Along the Simplon's steep and rugged road,
Following a band of muleteers, we reached
A halting-place, where all together took
Their noon-tide meal. Hastily rose our guide,
Leaving us at the board; awhile we lingered,
Then paced the beaten downward way that led
Right to a rough stream's edge, and there broke off;
The only track now visible was one   570
That from the torrent's further brink held forth
Conspicuous invitation to ascend
A lofty mountain. After brief delay
Crossing the unbridged stream, that road we took,
And clomb with eagerness, till anxious fears
Intruded, for we failed to overtake
Our comrades gone before. By fortunate chance,
While every moment added doubt to doubt,
A peasant met us, from whose mouth we learned
That to the spot which had perplexed us first   580
We must descend, and there should find the road,
Which in the stony channel of the stream
Lay a few steps, and then along its banks;
And, that our future course, all plain to sight,
Was downwards, with the current of that stream.
Loth to believe what we so grieved to hear,
For still we had hopes that pointed to the clouds,
We questioned him again, and yet again;
But every word that from the peasant's lips
Came in reply, translated by our feelings,   590
Ended in this,—'that we had crossed the Alps'.

Imagination—here the Power so called
Through sad incompetence of human speech,
That awful Power rose from the mind's abyss
Like an unfathered vapour that enwraps,
At once, some lonely traveller. I was lost;
Halted without an effort to break through;
But to my conscious soul I now can say—

"I recognise thy glory:" in such strength
Of usurpation, when the light of sense   600
Goes out, but with a flash that has revealed
The invisible world, doth greatness make abode,
There harbours; whether we be young or old,
Our destiny, our being's heart and home,
Is with infinitude, and only there;
With hope it is, hope that can never die,
Effort, and expectation, and desire,
And something evermore about to be.
Under such banners militant, the soul
Seeks for no trophies, struggles for no spoils   610
That may attest her prowess, blest in thoughts
That are their own perfection and reward,
Strong in herself and in beatitude
That hides her, like the mighty flood of Nile
Poured from his fount of Abyssinian clouds
To fertilise the whole Egyptian plain.

The melancholy slackening that ensued
Upon those tidings by the peasant given
Was soon dislodged. Downwards we hurried fast,
And, with the half-shaped road which we had missed,   620
Entered a narrow <u>chasm</u>. The brook and road
Were fellow-travellers in this gloomy strait,
And with them did we journey several hours
At a slow pace. The immeasurable height
Of woods decaying, never to be decayed,
The stationary blasts of waterfalls,
And in the narrow rent at every turn
Winds thwarting winds, bewildered and forlorn,
The torrents shooting from the clear blue sky,
The rocks that muttered close upon our ears   630
Black drizzling crags that spake by the way-side
As if a voice were in them, the sick sight
And giddy prospect of the raving stream,
The unfettered clouds and region of the Heavens,
Tumult and peace, the darkness and the light—
Were all like workings of one mind, the features
Of the same face, blossoms upon one tree;
Characters of the great Apocalypse,
The types and symbols of Eternity,
Of first, and last, and midst, and without end.   640

That night our lodging was a house that stood
Alone within the valley, at a point
Where, tumbling from aloft, a torrent swelled
The rapid stream whose margin we had trod;
A dreary mansion, large beyond all need,
With high and spacious rooms, deafened and stunned
By noise of waters, making innocent sleep
Lie melancholy among weary bones.

Uprisen betimes, our journey we renewed,
Led by the stream, ere noon-day magnified   650
Into a lordly river, broad and deep,
Dimpling along in silent majesty,
With mountains for its neighbours, and in view
Of distant mountains and their snowy tops,
And thus proceeding to Locarno's Lake,
Fit resting-place for such a visitant.
Locarno! spreading out in width like Heaven,
How dost thou cleave to the poetic heart,
Bask in the sunshine of the memory;
And Como! thou, a treasure whom the earth   660
Keeps to herself, confined as in a depth
Of Abyssinian privacy. I spake
Of thee, thy chestnut woods, and garden plots
Of Indian corn tended by dark-eyed maids;
Thy lofty steeps, and pathways roofed with vines,
Winding from house to house, from town to town,
Sole link that binds them to each other; walks,
League after league, and cloistral avenues,
Where silence dwells if music be not there:
While yet a youth undisciplined in verse,   670
Through fond ambition of that hour I strove
To chant your praise; nor can approach you now
Ungreeted by a more melodious Song,
Where tones of Nature smoothed by learned Art
May flow in lasting current. Like a breeze
Or sunbeam over your domain I passed
In motion without pause; but ye have left
Your beauty with me, a serene accord
Of forms and colours, passive, yet endowed
In their submissiveness with power as sweet   680
And gracious, almost, might I dare to say,
As virtue is, or goodness; sweet as love,
Or the remembrance of a generous deed,

Or mildest visitations of pure thought,
When God, the giver of all joy, is thanked
Religiously, in silent blessedness;
Sweet as this last herself, for such it is.

With those delightful pathways we advanced,
For two days' space, in presence of the Lake,
That, stretching far among the Alps, assumed   690
A character more stern. The second night,
From sleep awakened, and misled by sound
Of the church clock telling the hours with strokes
Whose import then we had not learned, we rose
By moonlight, doubting not that day was nigh,
And that meanwhile, by no uncertain path,
Along the winding margin of the lake,
Led, as before, we should behold the scene
Hushed in profound repose. We left the town
Of Gravedona with this hope; but soon   700
Were lost, bewildered among woods immense,
And on a rock sate down, to wait for day.
An open place it was, and overlooked,
From high, the sullen water far beneath,
On which a dull red image of the moon
Lay bedded, changing oftentimes its form
Like an uneasy snake. From hour to hour
We sate and sate, wondering, as if the night
Had been ensnared by witchcraft. On the rock
At last we stretched our weary limbs for sleep,   710
But 'could not' sleep, tormented by the stings
Of insects, which, with noise like that of noon,
Filled all the woods: the cry of unknown birds;
The mountains more by blackness visible
And their own size, than any outward light;
The breathless wilderness of clouds; the clock
That told, with unintelligible voice,
The widely parted hours; the noise of streams,
And sometimes rustling motions nigh at hand,
That did not leave us free from personal fear;   720
And, lastly, the withdrawing moon, that set
Before us, while she still was high in heaven;—
These were our food; and such a summer's night
Followed that pair of golden days that shed
On Como's Lake, and all that round it lay,
Their fairest, softest, happiest influence.

But here I must break off, and bid farewell
To days, each offering some new sight, or fraught
With some untried adventure, in a course
Prolonged till sprinklings of autumnal snow   730
Checked our unwearied steps. Let this alone
Be mentioned as a parting word, that not
In hollow exultation, dealing out
Hyperboles of praise comparative,
Not rich one moment to be poor for ever;
Not prostrate, overborne, as if the mind
Herself were nothing, a mere pensioner
On outward forms—did we in presence stand
Of that magnificent region. On the front
Of this whole Song is written that my heart   740
Must, in such Temple, needs have offered up
A different worship. Finally, whate'er
I saw, or heard, or felt, was but a stream
That flowed into a kindred stream; a gale,
Confederate with the current of the soul,
To speed my voyage; every sound or sight,
In its degree of power, administered
To grandeur or to tenderness,—to the one
Directly, but to tender thoughts by means
Less often instantaneous in effect;   750
Led me to these by paths that, in the main,
Were more circuitous, but not less sure
Duly to reach the point marked out by Heaven.

Oh, most beloved Friend! a glorious time,
A happy time that was; triumphant looks
Were then the common language of all eyes;
As if awaked from sleep, the Nations hailed
Their great expectancy: the fife of war
Was then a spirit-stirring sound indeed,
A blackbird's whistle in a budding grove.   760
We left the Swiss exulting in the fate
Of their near neighbours; and, when shortening fast
Our pilgrimage, nor distant far from home,
We crossed the Brabant armies on the fret
For battle in the cause of Liberty.
A stripling, scarcely of the household then
Of social life, I looked upon these things
As from a distance; heard, and saw, and felt,

Was touched, but with no intimate concern;
I seemed to move along them, as a bird   770
Moves through the air, or as a fish pursues
Its sport, or feeds in its proper element;
I wanted not that joy, I did not need
Such help; the ever-living universe,
Turn where I might, was opening out its glories,
And the independent spirit of pure youth
Called forth, at every season, new delights,
Spread round my steps like sunshine o'er green fields.

The Idiot and the Thorn

Wordsworth has an anthropological vision, as he is concerned with how human beings possess certain types of possibilities and limitations. This includes the world of marginal individuals, such as idiots and mad women, who provide him with an account of the progress of the human mind and its imagination—imagination steeped both in the comic and the profoundly tragic. Wordsworth's analysis of the community and the relationship of marginal individuals within these communities is a study worth exploring from a socio-poetic point of view; students can perceive the poet's view of idiots and female outcasts in society. In the narrative poems, "The Idiot Boy" and "The Thorn," Wordsworth explores the relationship of the marginal individual to the society that surrounds him.

My Commentary on "The Idiot Boy"

Wordsworth makes the Idiot a figure of mystery, stretching the limits of our understanding." The Idiot Boy" encompasses a general air of fuss, bother and comic confusion. In the poem, the reader is able to perceive of Wordsworth's noble conception of Idiots, "...that their life if hidden with God. They are worshipped, probably from a feeling of this sort, in several parts of the East. Among the Alps where they are numerous, they are considered I believe, as a blessing to the family to which they belong. The ever-changing point of view and the repetitive style of the ballad, combine to give the impression of hectic activity. By midnight, Betty is worried, and by one o'clock "she's in a sad quandary." Her excitability is contrasted with the figure of the doctor. When Betty knocks on his door, the doctor is a comic figure: The doctor at the casement shows,/ His glimmering eyes that peep and doze; And one hand rubs in old night-cap."

When he discovers what Betty wants, since she is too preoccupied with Johnny that she forgets to ask him to see Susan, the Doctor's comic character disappears as he states," What woman! should I know of him?" And, grumbling, he went back to bed." Since Betty has called on him in the middle of the night, it is understandable that the doctor is irritable. Yet his impatience, and his abrupt dismissal of Betty - "What woman!"- is of great significance to the poem. It is the voice of a man who knows his position in the community, whose brief appearance in the poem is a reminder of the features of society, which the poem is not about. The poem is not about a structured society, or about reasonable action; it is about an idiot and the human love that surrounds him.

As an idiot, Johnny stands outside normal experience. Johnny is not an outcast, as he has the best of both worlds. He is able to see further, to lead an imaginative and happy life, beyond the grasp of ordinary men; yet he also has the joy of being surrounded by human love. In the poem's community, strange and marvelous things happen: it is a world of natural intuitions, affections and spontaneous recovery from illness. By his rational conduct as a member of a structured society, the doctor cuts himself off from the happiness in which Johnny and Betty find the recovered Susan.

Four travelers, not three: in this world of natural happiness and love, the human and animal kingdoms are united in mutual joy. At this point Johnny, the divine fool, makes his only speech of the poem:

" And thus to Betty's question, he
Made answer, like a traveller bold,
(His very words I give to you,)
'The cocks did crow to-whoo, to-whoo,
And the sun did shine so cold.'
-Thus answered Johnny in his glory,
And that was all his traveller's story."

Johnny is in his glory: in one way, he is being led home after his night's adventures, surrounded by love and affection, and sitting on the pony he loves; in a deeper sense he is 'in his glory' because he has seen something marvelous and is able to capture it in words that are imaginative. He has seen the moon as a cold, shining sun; he has entered a world forever closed to the doctor. The poet is not allowed to describe what actually happened to Johnny, but the end of the poem gives the reader/listener a glimpse of the world that lies beyond the reach of reason and ordinary sense. Johnny's experience is obtained without the loss of human love. The poet acknowledges some inability on his part to pierce to the core of his nature and reaction to the world around him:

"I to the muses have been bound,
These fourteen years, by strong indentures;
Oh gentle muses!let me tell
But half of what to him befel
For sure he met with strange adventures."

In the "Idiot Boy," humor is a defense against the ominous threats facing Johnny. Anxiety is localized in his mother, Betty Foy, and her friend Susan Gale as part of the poetic strategy for displacing the real threats that faced an idiot displaced from his family. Wordsworth transforms the idiot into an exotic being, who held within his silence fundamental truths about human nature.

Betty Foy indulges in a romantic vision of her son as a quixotic hero on a quest and seeks to give him a lesson in horsemanship. Betty sees her son as a village hero, a figure in a romance. She repeats and repeats a carefully ordered set of instructions:

> "Both what to follow, what to shun
> What do, and what to leave undone,
> How turn to left, and how to right."

Throughout this lesson, Johnny has been brandishing his holly bough and shaking his head and the bridle, in a state bordering on ecstasy. Even his horse knows more than he; born with the innate knowledge that Johnny lacks-instincts-it thinks.

In keeping with her loving overestimation of her son's abilities, Betty attributes speech to him. She has no difficulty in understanding his "burr,burr,burr" as the noise he loves, a pure expression of joy:

> "And Johnny burrs, and laughs aloud;
> Whether in cunning or in joy
> I cannot tell; but while he laughs,
> Betty a drunken pleasure quaffs
> To hear again her Idiot Boy."

The basic function of the utterances in the joyful reunion is not to represent ideas, but to create **contact.** Talking is like touching, and the 'drunken pleasure' that Betty draws from hearing her son speak again is returned as she holds onto him tightly, kisses him "o'er and o'er again," cries and "pats the pony." The phrase "o'er and o'er again" recalls Betty's earlier attempt at pedagogy, it suggests that her assumption that her repeated instructions were understood as more than simply the loving touch of words. Johnny's strange adventures into the woods constitute an educational process that is set against Betty's failed pedagogy.

What of Susan Gale's strange disease and unusual cure? The doctor never arrives to give a diagnosis. Her illness can be seen as a comic device that occasions Johnny's mock epic quest. Eventually her mental terror is substituted for bodily pains:

"She turned and tossed in bed,
On all sides doubts and terrors met her;
Point after point she did discuss;
And, while her mind was fighting thus,
Her body still grew better.

"Alas!what is become of them?
These fears can never be endured;
I'll to the wood."-The word scarce said,
Did Susan rise up from her bed,
As if by magic cured."

"The Idiot Boy"

'Tis eight o'clock,—a clear March night,
The moon is up—the sky is blue,
The owlet in the moonlight air,
He shouts from nobody knows where;
He lengthens out his lonely shout,
Halloo! halloo! a long halloo!

—Why bustle thus about your door,
What means this bustle, Betty Foy?
Why are you in this mighty fret?
And why on horseback have you set
Him whom you love, your idiot boy?

Beneath the moon that shines so bright,
Till she is tired, let Betty Foy
With girt and stirrup fiddle-faddle;
But wherefore set upon a saddle
Him whom she loves, her idiot boy?

There's scarce a soul that's out of bed;
Good Betty! put him down again;
His lips with joy they burr at you,
But, Betty! what has he to do
With stirrup, saddle, or with rein?

The world will say 'tis very idle,
Bethink you of the time of night;
There's not a mother, no not one,
But when she hears what you have done,
Oh! Betty she'll be in a fright.

But Betty's bent on her intent,
For her good neighbour, Susan Gale,
Old Susan, she who dwells alone,
Is sick, and makes a piteous moan,
As if her very life would fail.

There's not a house within a mile,
No hand to help them in distress
Old Susan lies a bed in pain,
And sorely puzzled are the twain,
For what she ails they cannot guess.

And Betty's husband's at the wood,
Where by the week he doth abide,
A woodman in the distant vale;
There's none to help poor Susan Gale,
What must be done? what will betide?

And Betty from the lane has fetched
Her pony, that is mild and good,
Whether he be in joy or pain,
Feeding at will along the lane,
Or bringing faggots from the wood.

An he is all in traveling trim,
And by the moonlight, Betty Foy
Has up upon the saddle set,
The like was never heard of yet,
Him whom she loves, her idiot boy.

And he must post without delay
Across the bridge that's in the dale,
And by the church, and o'er the down,
To bring a doctor from the town,
Or she will die, old Susan Gale.

There is no need of boot or spur,
There is no need of whip or wand,
For Johnny has his holly-bough,
And with a hurly-burly now

He shakes the green bough in his hand.
And Betty o'er and o'er has told
The boy who is her best delight,

Both what to follow, what to shun,
What to do, and what to leave undone,
How to turn left, and how to right.

And Betty's most especial charge,
Was, "Johnny! Johnny! mind that you
"Come home again, nor stop at all,
"Come home again, whate'er befal,
"My Johnny do, I pray you do."

To this did Johnny answer make,
Both with his head, and with his hand,
And proudly shook the bridle too,
And then! his words were not a few,
Which Betty well could understand.

And now that Johnny is just going,
Though Betty's in a mighty flurry,
She gently pats the pony's side,
On which her idiot boy must ride,
And seems no longer in a hurry.

But when the pony moved his legs,
Oh! then for the poor idiot boy!
For joy he cannot hold the bridle,
For joy his head and heels are idle,
He's idle all for very joy.

And while the pony moves his legs,
In Johnny's left-hand you may see,
The green bough's motionless and dead;
The moon that shines above his head
Is not more still and mute than he.

His heart it was so full of glee,
That till full fifty yards were gone,
He quite forgot his holly whip,
And all his skill in horsemanship,
Oh! happy, happy, happy John.

And Betty's standing at the door,
And Betty's face with joy o'erflows,
Proud of herself, and proud of him,
She sees him in his traveling trim;
How quietly her Johnny goes.

The silence of her idiot boy,
What hope it sends to Betty's heart!
He's at the guide-post—he turns right,
She watches till he's out of sight,
And Betty will not then depart.

Burr, burr—now Johnny's lips they burr,
As loud as any mill, or near it,
Meek as a lamb the pony moves,
And Johnny makes the noise he loves,
And Betty listens, glad to hear it.

Away she hies to Susan Gale:
And Johnny's in a merry tune,
The owlets hoot, the owlets curr,
And Johnny's lips they burr, burr, burr,
And on he goes beneath the moon.

His steed and he right well agree,
For of this pony there's rumour,
That should he lose his eyes and ears,
And should he live a thousand years,
He never will be out of humour.

But then he is a horse that thinks!
And when he thinks his pace is slack;
Now, though he knows poor Johnny well,
Yet for his life he cannot tell
What he has got upon his back.

So through the moonlight lanes they go,
And far into the moonlight dale,
And by the church, and o'er the down,
To bring a doctor from the town,
To comfort poor old Susan Gale.

And Betty, now at Susan's side,
Is in the middle of her story,
What comfort Johnny soon will bring,
With many a most diverting thing,
Of Johnny's wit and Johnny's glory.

And Betty's still at Susan's side:
By this time she's not quite so flurried;

Demure with porringer and plate
She sits, as if in Susan's fate
Her life and soul were buried.

But Betty, poor good woman! she,
You plainly in her face may read it,
Could lend out of that moment's store
Five years of happiness or more,
To any that might need it.

But yet I guess that now and then
With Betty all was not so well,
And to the road she turns her ears,
And thence full many a sound she hears,
Which she to Susan will not tell.

Poor Susan moans, poor Susan groans,
"As sure as there's a moon in heaven,"
Cries Betty, "he'll be back again;
"They'll both be here, 'tis almost ten,
"They'll both be here before eleven."

Poor Susan moans, poor Susan groans,
The clock gives warning for eleven;
'Tis on the stroke—"If Johnny's near,"
Quoth Betty "he will soon be here,
"As sure as there's a moon in heaven."

The clock is on the stroke of twelve,
And Johnny is not yet in sight,
The moon's in heaven, as Betty sees,
But Betty is not quite at ease;
And Susan has a dreadful night.

And Betty, half an hour ago,
On Johnny vile reflections cast;
"A little idle sauntering thing!"
With other names, an endless string,
But now that time is gone and past.

And Betty's drooping at the heart,
That happy time all past and gone,
"How can it be he is so late?
"The doctor he has made him wait,
"Susan! they'll both be here anon."

And Susan's growing worse and worse,
And Betty's in sad quandary;
And then there's nobody to say
If she must go or she must stay:
—She's in a sad quandary.

The clock is on the stroke of one;
But neither Doctor nor his guide
Appear along the moonlight road
There's neither horse nor man abroad,
And Betty's still at Susan's side.

And Susan she begins to fear
Of sad mischances not a few,
That Johnny may perhaps be drown'd,
Or lost perhaps, and never found;
Which they must both for ever rue.

She prefaced half a hint of this
With, "God forbid it should be true!"
At the first word that Susan said
Cried Betty, rising from the bed,
"Susan, I'd gladly stay with you.

"I must be gone, I must away.
"Consider, Johnny's but half-wise;
"Susan, we must take care of him,
"If he is hurt in life or limb" —
"Oh God forbid!" poor Susan cries.

"What can I do?" says Betty, going,
"What can I do to ease your pain?
"Good Susan tell me, and I'll stay;
"I fear you're in a dreadful way,
"But I shall soon be back again."

"Good Betty go, good Betty go,
"There's nothing that can ease my pain."
Then off she hies, but with a prayer
That God poor Susan's life would spare,
Till she comes back again.

So, through the moonlight lane she goes,
And far into the moonlight dale;

And how she ran, and how she walked,
And all that to herself she talked,
Would surely be a tedious tale.

In high and low, above, below,
In great and small, in round and square,
In tree and tower was Johnny seen,
In bush and brake, in black and green,
'Twas Johnny, Johnny, every where.

She's past the bridge that's in the dale,
And now the thought torments her sore,
Johnny perhaps his horse forsook,
To hunt the moon that's in the brook,
And never will be heard of more.

And now she's high upon the down,
Alone amid a prospect wide;
There's neither Johnny nor his horse,
Among the fern or in the gorse;
There's neither doctor nor his guide.

"Oh saints! what is become of him?
"Perhaps he's climbed into an oak,
"Where he will stay till he is dead;
"Or sadly he has been misled,
And joined the wandering gypsey-folk.

"Or him that wicked pony's carried
"To the dark cave, the goblin's hall,
"Or in the castle he's pursuing,
"Among the ghosts, his own undoing;
"Or playing with the waterfall."

At poor old Susan then she railed,
While to the town she posts away;
"If Susan had not been so ill,
"Alas! I should have had him still,
"My Johnny, till my dying day."

Poor Betty! in this sad distemper,
The doctor's self would hardly spare,
Unworthy things she talked and wild,
Even he, of cattle the most mild,
The pony had his share.

And now she's got into the town,
And to the doctor's door she hies;
'Tis silence all on every side;
The town so long, the town so wide,
Is silent as the skies.

And now she's at the doctor's door,
She lifts the knocker, rap, rap, rap,
The doctor at the casement shews,
His glimmering eyes that peep and doze;
And one hand rubs his old night-cap.

"Oh Doctor! Doctor! where's my Johnny?"
"I'm here, what is't you want with me?"
"Oh Sir! you know I'm Betty Foy,
"And I have lost my poor dear boy,
"You know him—him you often see;

"He's not as wise as some folks be,"
"The devil take his wisdom!" said
The Doctor, looking somewhat grim,
"What, woman! should I know of him?"
And, grumbling, he went back to bed.

"O woe is me! O woe is me!
"here will I die; here will I die;
"I thought to find my Johnny here,
"But he is neither far nor near,
"Oh! what a wretched mother I!"

She stops, she stands, she looks about,
Which way to turn she cannot tell.
Poor Betty! it would ease her pain
If she had the heart to knock again;
—The clock strikes three—a dismal knell!

Then up along the town she hies,
No wonder if her senses fail,
This piteous news so much it shock'd her,
She quite forgot to send the Doctor,
To comfort poor old Susan Gale.

And now she's high upon the down,
And she can see a mile of road,

"Oh cruel! I'm almost three-score;
"Such night as this was ne'er before,
"There's not a single soul abroad."

She listens, but she cannot hear
The foot of horse, the voice of man;
The streams with softest sound are flowing,
The grass you almost hear it growing,
You hear it now if e'er you can.

The owlets through the long blue night
Are shouting to each other still:
Fond lovers, yet not quite hob nob,
They lengthen out the tremulous sob,
That echoes far from hill to hill.

Poor Betty now has lost all hope,
Her thoughts are bent on deadly sin;
A green-grown pond she just has pass'd,
And from the brink she hurries fast,
Lest she should drown herself therein.

And now she sits her down and weeps;
Such tears she never shed before;
"Oh dear, dear pony! my sweet joy!
"Oh carry back my idiot boy!
"And we will ne'er o'erload thee more."

A thought is come into her head;
"The pony he is mild and good,
"And we have always used him well;
"Perhaps he's gone along the dell,
"And carried Johnny to the wood."

Then up she springs as if on wings;
She thinks no more of deadly sin;
If Betty fifty ponds should see,
The last of all her thoughts would be,
To drown herself therein.

Oh reader! now that I might tell
What Johnny and his horse are doing!
What they've been doing all this time,
Oh could I put it into rhyme,
A most delightful tale pursuing!

Perhaps, and no unlikely thought!
He with his pony now doth roam
The cliffs and peaks so high that are,
To lay his hands upon a star,
And in his pocket bring it home.

Perhaps he's turned himself about,
His face unto his horse's tail,
And still and mute, in wonder lost,
All like a silent horseman-ghost,
He travels on along the vale.

And now, perhaps, he's hunting sheep,
A fierce and dreadful hunter he!
Yon valley, that's so trim and green,
In five months' time, should he be seen,
A desart wilderness will be.

Perhaps, with head and heels on fire,
And like the very soul of evil,
He's galloping away, away,
And so he'll gallop on for aye,
The bane of all that dread the devil.

I to the muses have been bound,
These fourteen years, by strong indentures;
Oh gentle muses! let me tell
But half of what to him befel,
For sure he met with strange adventures.

Oh gentle muses! Is this kind?
Why will ye thus my suit repel?
Why of your further aid bereave me?
And can you thus unfriended leave me?
Ye muses! whom I love so well.

Who's yon, that, near the waterfall,
Which thunders down with headlong force,
Beneath the moon, yet shining fair,
As careless as if nothing were,
Sits upright on a feeding horse?

Unto his horse, that's feeding free,
He seems, I think, the reins to give;

Of moon or stars he takes no heed;
Of such we in romances read,
—'Tis Johnny! Johnny! as I live.

And that's the very pony, too.
Where is she, where is Betty Foy?
She hardly can sustain her fears;
The roaring water-fall she hears,
And cannot find her idiot boy.

Your pony's worth his weight in gold,
Then calm your terrors, Betty Foy!
She's coming from among the trees,
And now, all full in view, she sees
Him whom she loves, her idiot boy.

And Betty sees the pony too:
Why stand you thus Good Betty Foy?
It is no goblin, 'tis no ghost,
'Tis he whom you so long have lost,
He whom you love, your idiot boy.

She looks again—her arms are up—
She screams—she cannot move for joy;
She darts as with a torrent's force,
She has almost o'erturned the horse,
And fast she holds her idiot boy.

And Johnny burrs and laughs aloud,
Whether in cunning or in joy,
I cannot tell; but while he laughs,
Betty a drunken pleasure quaffs,
To hear again her idiot boy.

And now she's at the pony's tail,
And now she's at the pony's head,
On that side now, and now on this,
And almost stifled with her bliss,
A few sad tears does Betty shed.

She kisses o'er and o'er again,
Him whom she loves, her idiot boy,
She's happy here, she's happy there,
She is uneasy every where:
Her limbs are all alive with joy.

She pats the pony, where or when
She knows not, happy Betty Foy!
The little pony glad may be,
But he is milder far than she,
You hardly can perceive his joy.

"Oh! Johnny, never mind the Doctor;
"You've done your best, and that is all."
She took the reins, when this was said,
And gently turned the pony's head
From the loud water-fall.

By this the stars were almost gone,
The moon was setting on the hill,
So pale you scarcely looked at her:
The little birds began to stir,
Though yet their tongues were still.

The pony, Betty, and her boy,
Wind slowly through the windy dale:
And who is she, be-times abroad,
That hobbles up the steep rough road?
Who is it, but old Susan Gale?

Long Susan lay deep lost in thought,
And many dreadful fears beset her,
Both for her messenger and nurse;
And as her mind grew worse and worse,
Her body it grew better.

She turned, she toss'd herself in bed,
On all sides doubts and terrors met her;
Point after point did she discuss;
And while her mind was fighting thus,
Her body still grew better.

"Alas! what is become of them?
"These fears can never be endured,
"I'll to the wood."—The word scarce said
Did Susan rise up from her bed,
As if by magic cured.

Away she posts up hill and down,
And to the wood at length is come,

She pies her friends, she shouts a greeting;
Oh me! it is a merry meeting,
As ever was in Christendom.

The owls have hardly sung their last,
While our four travelers homeward wend;
The owls have hooted all night long,
And with the owls began my song,
And with the owls must end.

For while they all were travelling home,
Cried Betty, "Tell us, Johnny, do,
"Where all this long night you have been,
"What you have heard, what you have seen,
"And Johnny, mind you tell us true."

Now Johnny all night long had heard
The owls in tuneful concert strive;
No doubt too he the moon had seen;
For in the moon light he had been
From eight o'clock till five.

And thus to Betty's question, he
Made answer, like a traveller bold,
(His very words I give to you,)
"The cocks did crow to-whoo, tu-whoo,
"And the sun did shine so cold."

—Thus answered Johnny in his glory,
And that was all his travel's story.

My Commentary on "The Thorn"

"The Thorn" is the contrasting opposite of "The Idiot Boy." Instead of celebrating insight and community, it confronts the problems of betrayal, separation and despair. Although there are certain shared qualities - the ballad style, the central figure who is mad, the intrusive narrator -these only serve to emphasize the contrasts between Johnny, lapped in the warmth of Betty's love, and Martha Ray, sitting alone on the mountain. The contrast is between Johnny sitting alone on the pony `in his glory' and the huddled figure by the thorn, while the thorn itself is used as a symbol of stunted growth:

It looks so old and grey.
Not higher than a two-years' child,
It stands erect this aged thorn;
No leaves it has, no thorny points;
It is a mass of knotted joints,
A wretched thing forlorn.

The mixture of the child's stature with the old and grey appearance of the bush suggests a grotesque mixture of youth and age, and a stunted life. It is a prey to parasites:

Like rock or stone, it is o'ergrown
With lichens to the very top,
And hung with heavy tufts of moss,
A melancholy crop:
Up from the earth those mosses creep,
And this poor thorn they clasp it round
So close, you'd say that they were bent
With plain and manifest intent,
To drag it to the ground.

The picture is one of natural misery, of one organism preying upon another. The thorn is barren, stunted, imprisoned, under attack from mosses and other hostile organisms. The woman who sits beside the thorn has many resemblances: she is barren by the loss of her baby, and stunted emotionally by the betrayal of Stephen Hill; as the moss tries to drag down the thorn, so the villagers censure Martha and try to bring her to justice; as the thorn has to withstand the winter gales, so Martha has to withstand the fierce breath of public opinion. As the thorn is 'bound' so Martha is also imprisoned, locked in a fixation of her own grief. She has a compulsive need to remain beside the thorn.

And all times of the day and night
This wretched woman thither goes,
And she is known to every star,
And every wind that blows.

The stars and the winds are free in comparison to the woman who is obsessed with one place and one idea. She is chained to the thorn, as the thorn is bound by the moss. She is stagnant as Johnny is a wanderer. "Oh misery! oh misery!/Oh woe is me! Oh misery!" is the refrain, Martha's only speech in the poem. She is fixated and obsessed. All her normal energies and happiness have been obstructed and retarded. We learn about Martha from the narrator. Here is a superstitious narrator rather than the animated narrator; the narrator is very much the observer rather than part of the storyteller. He accumulates information and knows about measurements and spaces: " I've measured it from side to side: /"'Tis three feet long, and two feet wide." The narrator makes no attempt to establish a relationship with the woman, but remains isolated. This is made clear when the sea-captain is caught in the mist and rain:

Instead of jutting crag, I found
A woman seated on the ground.
I did not speak-I saw her face,
Her face it was enough for me;

Martha remains the figure sitting on the ground, unaffected by his arrival. The lack of communication is her fault as much as it is his: she is obsessed by her grief, and he is frightened by her appearance.

The community is interested in Martha Ray, but only as a subject for speculation: they notice when she is pregnant, and farmer Simpson notices her calmness at the time of the child's birth; after that all is rumor:

some will say
She hanged her baby on the tree,
Some say she drowned it in the pond,
Which is a little step beyond,
But all and each agree,
The little babe was buried there,
Beneath that hill of moss so fair.

The whole idea of child-murder has an air of nasty speculation by the ignorant and the insensitive. They intend to find the evidence by digging up the baby, and the imagery of the spade seeking for the tiny bones is brutal and horrifying. They are repulsed by nature, as the grass quivers around them serving to emphasize the cruelty and insensitivity of man. The final image is not of the little hill of moss with its lively colors, but of the stunted thorn, and the woman sitting alone. To increase her misery and madness, she has lost her child by miscarriage or stillbirth. It is significant that though these villagers suspect Martha Ray, they never legally accuse her. When the villagers begin to dig for proof, " instantly the hill of moss/before their eyes began to stir!" Fearful of what this sight might portend, they decide to let matters stand. Though Martha Ray has escaped legal prosecution, there is nothing optimistic about the conclusion of the poem. She remains ostracized from the community and a continual object of fear, hostility, gossip, and debate.

The conflict and uncertainty are manifested in the mind and language of the narrator. When climbing among the hills, when the old sailor first came to the seaside village, he was caught in a terrible storm. Seeking a rock for shelter he came upon an isolated woman. "Instead of a jutting crag, I found/ A Woman seated on the ground." The narrator vascillates between two systems of explanation. He is unable to separate what he originally saw from its subsequent reconstruction in memory. The narrator, apart from describing her scarlet cloak, does not describe Martha Ray.

"The Thorn"

I

There is a thorn; it looks so old,
In truth you'd find it hard to say,
How it could ever have been young,
It looks so old and grey.
Not higher than a two-year's child,
It stands erect this aged thorn;
No leaves it has, no thorny points;
It is a mass of knotted joints,
A wretched thing forlorn.
It stands erect, and like a stone
With lichens it is overgrown.

II

Like rock or stone, it is o'ergrown
With lichens to the very top,
And hung with heavy tufts of moss,
A melancholy crop:
Up from the earth these mosses creep,
And this poor thorn they clasp it round
So close, you'd say that they were bent
With plain and manifest intent,
To drag it to the ground;
And all had joined in one endeavour
To bury this poor thorn for ever.

III

High on a mountain's highest ridge,
Where oft the stormy winter gale
Cuts like a scythe, while through the clouds
It sweeps from vale to vale;
Not five yards from the mountain-path,
This thorn you on your left espy;
And to the left, three yards beyond,
You see a little muddy pond
Of water, never dry;
I've measured it from side to side:
'Tis three feet long, and two feet wide.

IV

And close beside this aged thorn,
There is a fresh and lovely sight,
A beauteous heap, a hill of moss,
Just half a foot in height.
All lovely colours there you see.
All colours that were ever seen,
And mossy network too is there,
As if by hand of lady fair
The work had woven been,
And cups, the darlings of the eye,
So deep is their vermilion dye.

V

Ah me! what lovely tints are there!
Of olive-green and scarlet bright,
In spikes, in branches, and in stars,
Green, red, and pearly white.
This heap of earth o'ergrown with moss,
Which close beside the thorn you see,
So fresh in all its beauteous dyes,
As like as like can be:
But never, never any where,
An infant's grave was half so fair.

VI

Now would you see this aged thorn,
This pond and beauteous hill of moss,
You must take care and chuse your time
The mountain when to cross.
For oft there sits, between the heap
That's like an infant's grave in size,
And that same pond of which I spoke,
A woman in a scarlet cloak,
And to herself she cries,
"Oh misery! Oh misery!
"Oh woe is me! oh misery!"

VII

At all times of the day and night
This wretched woman thither goes,

And she is known to every star,
And every wind that blows;
And there beside the thorn she sits
When the blue day-light's in the skies,
And when the whirlwind's on the hill,
Or frosty air is keen and still,
And to herself she cries,
"Oh misery! oh misery!
"Oh woe is me! oh misery!"

VIII

"Now wherefore thus, by day and night,
"In rain, in tempest, and in snow,
"Thus to the dreary mountain-top
"Does this poor woman go?
"And why sits she beside the thorn
"When the blue day-light's in the sky,
"Or when the whirlwind's on the hill,
"Or frosty air is keen and still,
"And wherefore does she cry?—
"Oh wherefore" wherefore? tell me why
"Does she repeat that doleful cry?"

IX

I cannot tell; I wish I could;
For the true reason no one knows,
But if you'd gladly view the spot,
The spot to which she goes;
The heap that's like an infant grave,
The pond—and thorn, so old and grey,
Pass by her door—tis seldom shut—
And if you see her in her hut,
Then to the spot away!—
I never heard of such as dare
Approach the spot when she is there.

X

"But wherefore to the mountain-top
"Can this unhappy woman go,
"Whatever star is in the skies,
"Whatever wind may blow?"

Nay rack your brain—'tis all in vain,
I'll tell you every thing I know;
But to the thorn, and to the pond
Which is a little step beyond,
I wish that you would go:
Perhaps when you are at the place
You something of her tale may trace.

XI

I'll give you the best help I can:
Before you up the mountain go,
Up to the dreary mountain-top,
I'll tell you all I know.
'Tis now some two and twenty years,
Since she (her name is Martha Ray)
Gave with a maiden's true good will
Her company to Stephen Hill;
And she was blithe and gay,
And she was happy, happy still
Whene'er she thought of Stephen Hill.

XII

And they had fix'd the wedding-day,
The morning that must wed them both;
But Stephen to another maid
Had sworn another oath;
And with this other maid to church
Unthinking Stephen went—
Poor Martha! on that woful day
A cruel, cruel fire, they say,
Into her bones was sent:
It dried her body like a cinder,
And almost turn'd her brain to tinder.

XIII

They say, full six months after this,
While yet the summer-leaves were green,
She to the mountain-top would go,
And there was often seen.
'Tis said, a child was in her womb,
As now to any eye was plain;

She was with child, and she was mad,
Yet often she was sober sad
From her exceeding pain.
Oh me! ten thousand times I'd rather
That he had died, that cruel father!

XIV

Sad case for such a brain to hold
Communion with a stirring child!
Sad case, as you may think, for one
Who had a brain so wild!
Last Christmas when we talked of this,
Old Farmer Simpson did maintain,
That in her womb the infant wrought
About its mother's heart, and brought
Her senses back again:
And when at last, her time drew near,
Her looks were calm, her senses clear.

XV

No more I know, I wish I did,
And I would tell it all to you;
For what became of this poor child
There's none that ever knew:
And if a child was born or no,
There's no one that could ever tell;
And if 'twas born alive or dead,
There's no one knows, as I have said,
But some remember well,
That Martha Ray about this time
Would up the mountain often climb.

XVI

And all that winter, when at night
The wind blew from the mountain-peak,
'Twas worth your while, though in the dark,
The church-yard path to seek:
For many a time and oft were heard
Cries coming from the mountain-head,
Some plainly living voices were,
And others, I've heard many swear,

Were voices of the dead:
I cannot think, whate'er they say,
They had to do with Martha Ray.

XVII

But that she goes to this old thorn,
The thorn which I've described to you,
And there sits in a scarlet cloak,
I will be sworn is true.
For one day with my telescope,
To view the ocean wide and bright,
When to this country first I came,
Ere I had heard of Martha's name,
I climbed the mountain's height:
A storm came on, and I could see
No object higher than my knee.

XVIII

Twas mist and rain, and storm and rain,
No screen, no fence could I discover,
And then the wind! in faith, it was
A wind full ten times over.
I looked around, I thought I saw
A jutting crag, and off I ran,
Head-foremost, through the driving rain,
The shelter of the crag to gain,
And, as I am a man,
Instead of jutting crag, I found
A woman seated on the ground.

XIX

I did not speak—I saw her face,
Her face it was enough for me;
I turned about and heard her cry,
"O misery! O misery!"
And there she sits, until the moon
Through half the clear blue sky will go,
And when the little breezes make
The waters of the pond to shake,
As all the country know,
She shudders and you hear her cry,
"Oh misery! oh misery!

XX

"But what's the thorn? and what's the pond?
"And what's the hill of moss to her?
"And what's the creeping breeze that comes
"The little pond to stir?"
I cannot tell; but some will say
he hanged her baby on the tree,
Some say she drowned it in the pond,
Which is a little step beyond,
But all and each agree,
The little babe was buried there,
Beneath that hill of moss so fair.

XXI

I've heard the scarlet moss is red
With drops of that poor infant's blood;
But kill a new-born infant thus!
I do not think she could.
Some say, if to the pond you go,
And fix on it a steady view,
The shadow of a babe you trace,
A baby and a baby's face,
And that it looks at you;
Whene'er you look on it, 'tis plain
The baby looks at you again.

XXII

And some had sworn an oath that she
Should be to public justice brought;
And for the little infant's bones
With spades they would have sought.
But then the beauteous hill of moss
Before their eyes began to stir;
And for full fifty yards around,
The grass it shook upon the ground;
But all do still aver
The little babe is buried there,
Beneath that hill of moss so fair.

XXIII

I cannot tell how this may be,
But plain it is, the thorn is bound

With heavy tufts of moss, that strive
To drag it to the ground.
And this I know, full many a time,
When she was on the mountain high,
By day, and in the silent night,
When all the stars shone clear and bright,
That I have heard her cry,
"Oh misery! Oh misery!
"O woe is me! oh misery!"

Section **IV**

Satirists

Some of my favorite post-modern satirists include Bill Mahr and Jon Stewart; their work is easily accessible and widely read. I am including a few of my essays on centuries old satirists, who have been largely ignored in recent times.

4.a. My Commentary on *The Trimmer*
by George Saville, First Marquis of Halifax (1633-1695)

The Aristotelian Trimmer

Although Halifax's writings are bare of classical allusion, they are steeped in the influence of the Stagirite. " The Character of a Trimmer, " a frank and full confession of

Halifax's own political conviction, is a plea for moderation. The discourse of the character of the Trimmer, while never directly referenced within the teachings of Aristotelian influence, is clearly based on the philosophy of the mean teaching by example, an indisputably Aristotelian doctrine.

As Aristotle believed that all good actions possess a common characteristic, namely, a certain order or proportion, with virtue as a desirable mean between the extremes of "excess" and "defect," so also The Trimmer states that ,"... true vertue hath ever been thought to be a Trimmer, and to have its dwelling in the middle between the two Extreams" (Saville 103). The Aristotelian mean between two extremes exist as a boundary between vices, one vice characterized by " excess," the second vice distinguished through a "defect." For example, an excess of generosity would be considered as prodigality, while the defect of stinginess would be illiberality. The virtue of liberality exists as the mean between these two vices. The general principle of Aristotle is that rational insight always finds the right mean between the unreasonable extremes to which the natural impulsive life might lead. For example, the virtue of courage is the balanced mean between cowardice and rashness.

The Aristotelian doctrine of the mean was not proposed to exalt intellectual or behavioral mediocrity within the moral context of virtue. This " golden mean " does not resemble the mathematical mean in that it is not an exact average of two precisely calculable extremes. This mean is only discovered through a flexible mind that has matured through reason.

This doctrine of the mean appears in the Trimmer's philosophy, where political passions are not vices in themselves, but the raw material which could lead to either an "excess" or a " defect" in political vices, as they function either in disproportion through " excess " and " defect, " ¼ or in harmony through the balanced mean. Political harmony is at the core of the Trimmer's political philosophy. Confirmed by rationality and a balanced politics of compromise and moderation , the Trimmer rebukes excessive political passions as he states, " If (men's) passions are provoked, they being as much a part of us as our limbs, they lead men into a short way of arguing, that admitteth no distinction, and from the foundation of self-defense they will draw inferences that will have miserable effects upon the quiet of a government" (Saville 102). Irrational and excessive political passion, on the part of a few, is able to dissemble a well-ordered government, leading to extreme partisanship and revolutionary tremors, political factors based in argumentation rather then rationality.

In as much as the Aristotelian doctrine of the mean had an obvious influence on Halifax's writing " The Character of a Trimmer," Aristotle's impact upon the character of the Trimmer did not cease within that one theoretical principle. The Trimmer also appears to be a firm believer in the natural authority of the governing class. " If it be true that the wisest men make the laws, it is as true that the strongest do often interpret them; and as rivers belong as much to the channel wherein they run as to the spring from which they first rise, so the laws depend as much upon the pipes through which they are to pass, as upon the fountain from which they flow." Aristotle's doctrine is that men differ in intellectual and physical capabilities and are thereby qualified for different positions within society. The Trimmer strengthens this social structural position when he reminds the reader that even the conquered have paid homage to their new masters and obeyed their laws, recognizing by acquiescence the conqueror's power and authority to rule.

Aristotle believed that human nature, or shall we say the human average, is nearer to the beast than to the god. He believed that the great majority of men are " natural dunces and sluggards." He further postulates that, in any system whatever, these men sink to the bottom. Aristotle asserts, " From the hour of their birth some are marked for subjection, and others for command." Aristotle theorizes that some men know instinctively that they are born to greatness, to be a ruling authority, while at the same time he relegates those, who can only work with their hands, those lacking proficiency in intellectual gifts, to be slaves by natural order. Thus, all inferiors should be ruled by a master. Neither the Trimmer nor Aristotle are believers in social equality.

With reference to " Laws " and the state, both The Trimmer and Aristotle are of one mind. The Trimmer has " great veneration for laws in general." He contends that laws exist in the state to tie up the " beast" in man, for otherwise mankind would live in a state of " barbarism and hostility." Aristotle affirms that the state exists for an end, and this end is the supreme good of mankind, his moral and intellectual life. " It is evident that the state is a creature of nature, and that man is by nature a political animal. And he who by nature and not by mere accident is without a State, is either above humanity or below it... He who is unable to live in society, or who has no need because he is sufficient for himself, must be either a beast or a god."

Both political theorists agree that not only do laws subdue the beastly passions of men, but that these laws are naturally structured within the construction of an ordered state. All laws "flow from nature" and what does not come from nature is imposed by man. Civilized people must willingly submit to law. The Trimmer expounds on the natural laws of the state when he states that laws "...are to mankind that which the sun is to plants." Laws protect man from man. " Our laws are Trimmers, between the excess of unbounded Power, and the Extravagance of Liberty not enough restrained."

The power of the law, according to Aristotle, is meant to secure observance of the law, to maintain a balance of power, and therefore to maintain political stability. However, he also warns that " ...to pass lightly from old laws to new ones is a certain means of weakening the inmost essence of all law whatever." The Trimmer couldn't agree more, as he says, " To see the laws mangled, disguised, speak quite another language than their own, to see them thrown from the dignity of protecting mankind, to the disgraceful office of destroying them...will raise men's anger above the power of laying it down again."

The Trimmer believes in the natural law, " innocent and uncorrupted nature." It is only in the state that man can live the good life, and since the good life is man's natural end, the state must be called a natural society.

Aristotle believes that a government is good when it aims at the good of the whole community, bad when it cares only for itself. Aristotle lists three types of governments, which are good: monarchy, aristocracy, and constitutional government or " polity." By contrast, there are three forms of less desirable governments: tyranny, oligarchy and democracy. Good and bad governments, in Aristotelian terms, are defined by the ethical qualities of the holders of power, and not specifically by the form of constitution. Aristotle holds, in accordance with the golden mean, that leaders with " moderate competence "...are most likely to be associated with virtue, founding a reestablishment of the golden mean in terms of the temperament of leadership and authority.

The Trimmer also enunciates a political philosophy of considerable flexibility and moderation with regard to the temperament of leadership - a politics of the possible, a philosophy based upon principles of honesty, tolerance, and above all, affection. Where Aristotle stressed the virtue of moderate competence, the Trimmer emphasizes the virtue of a loving ruler.

"He who feareth the king, only because he can punish, must wish there were no king; so that without a principle of love, there can be no true allegiance, and there must remain perpetual seeds of resistance against a power that is built upon such an unnatural foundation, as that of fear and terror." The Trimmer here establishes the virtue of love as a mean between fear and terror.

In tune with the Trimmer, Aristotle believed that the presupposition for moral actions, on the part of citizens, is freedom, including freedom from oppression. Since man cannot be forced into political responsibility, he must be invited to incur this responsibility voluntarily. If a man is politically forced to act under physical coercion (fear and terror), or if he acts in ignorance, he cannot be held responsible for his political actions by the ruling authority.

The union of the ruler and the ruled is an inviolable bond, according to the Trimmer. The idea of the king and the kingdom are inseparable. The king is head of the law, and "...is superior by his Vertue." However, to inspire citizens to participate voluntarily in politics, citizens must understand that "... Laws are jewels...nowhere better set, than in the constitution of our English government, if rightly understood, and carefully preserved." The Trimmer considers that rulers must possess dignity, so that public contempt will be in check. Rulers must not "...impose an abject and sordid servility...When a despotic Prince hath bruised all his subjects with a slavish obedience, all the force he uses cannot subdue his own fears." From the Trimmer's point of view, it is impossible for rulers to do injustice and not to fear revenge.

With regard to the stable and secure possession of authority and leadership by Kings and rulers, Aristotle's influence on the Trimmer is obvious. The Trimmer first emphasizes that Princes must be moderate in their quest for power. " In power," he states, " the way for princes to keep it, is not to grasp more than their arms can hold." The Trimmer also warns that a Prince must be jealous of his power, and advises not to disperse this power to others who could eventually eclipse him. Also, it is inadvisable for a Prince to allow those who advise him to lead him, as he would then become a rival against those to whom he has parceled out favor. While the Trimmer more specifically addresses this advise to a monarch, Aristotle addresses similar advice to tyrants. In a distinctly Machiavellian tone, Aristotle explains what a tyrant must do to retain power. He must prevent the rise of any person of exceptional merit, either by execution or by assassination.

The Trimmer holds a balanced opinion towards a constitutional monarchy, a form of government he perceives as both moderate and objectively workable. Although the Trimmer expresses that he " ...owneth a passion for liberty, " he explains that this passion is deliberately restrained, so that it does not interfere with his being loyal to the crown. He further asserts that the idea of "liberty" can be seductive to the maddening crowd. " Liberty", he states, " is the mistress of mankind," dazzling us with her charms so that men run after her. In order to achieve a balance of power, and to find a compromise between absolute liberty and the natural authority of Princes, the Trimmer reckons that it is within the " blessed constitution " where "...dominion and liberty are reconciled... The crown hath power sufficient to protect our liberties. The people have so much liberty as is necessary to make them useful to the crown."

The Trimmer engages in the Aristotelian debate over which is better, a monarchy or a commonwealth: " Monarchy, a thing that leaveth men no liberty, and a commonwealth, such a one as alloweth them no quiet." The Trimmer, philosophically influenced by the golden mean, desires to compromise between what he considers to be two extreme forms of government. Although the Trimmer acknowledges that Monarchy is generally loved by the people for its ceremonial pomp, he also admits that it can never be perfect and absolute. A Monarch must achieve a reasonable moderation of power. " If the will of a Prince is contrary either to reason itself, or to the universal opinion of his subjects, the law by a kind of restraint rescueth him from a disease that would undo him; if his will on the other side is reasonable and well-directed, that will immediately becometh a law, and he is arbitrary by an easy and natural consequence, without taking pains, or overturning the world for it."

Aristotle, although acknowledging a monarchy to be a desirable form of government, believed that the best practical " polity " would be an aristocracy, which he considered to be the rule of the informed and capable few. " For a right election can only be made by those who have knowledge: a geometrician, e.g. will choose rightly in matters of geometry; or a pilot in matters of navigation."

Both political philosophers agree that a democracy is usually a revolt through revolution against plutocracy. Although Aristotle acknowledges that this " rule by the poor " has some advantages, namely, that "...the people, though individually they may be worse judges than those who have special knowledge, are collectively as good." Yet democracy, for Aristotle, is on the whole inferior to aristocracy, for it is based upon a false assumption of equality. Aristotle concludes that the ballot should be limited to the intelligent, because the mass of people are so easily misled and so fickle in both their political views and their political loyalties. What Aristotle suggests is a combination of democracy and aristocracy. Constitutional government offers this happy union, and the Trimmer could not be in greater accord with this Aristotelian theory.

While discussing various types of constitutions, Aristotle divides governments into those who aim at the common interest and those who aim at their own private interest. For Aristotle, the political ideal is that one man should so transcend all the other citizens individually, with respect to intellectual excellence, that he would be the natural ruler or monarch. Realistically, of course, the perfect man does not appear, and thus aristocracy, the rule of many good men, is considered by Aristotle to be a more practical realization of government than monarchy. However, he also recognizes that even an aristocracy is perhaps too high an ideal for the modern state, and so advocates "polity", in which "there naturally exists a warlike multitude able to obey and to rule in turn by a law which gives office to the well-to-do according to their desert." Whatever type of constitution is constructed, Aristotle warns that it must be careful not to go to extremes; for if either a democracy or an oligarchy is pushed to extremes, the ensuing rise of malcontented political coalitions would be sure to result in a revolution.

The Trimmer states that he is a friend to all parliaments, despite their excesses and faults, and however troublesome they may be to a political administration. However, being a true compromiser and believer in the natural authority of rulers, he qualifies these remarks by also proclaiming that no government is perfect "...except a kind of Omnipotence reside in it, to exercise upon great occasions. Now this cannot be obtained by force alone upon the people, let it never be so great, there must be their consent too, or else a nation moveth only by being driven, a sluggish and constrained motion, void of that life and vigour which is necessary to produce great things..." Aristotle also considered it essential that the citizen sit in the Assembly and in the Law Courts, as, in his view, citizens should take their share in ruling and being ruled by turn.

The Trimmer believes in the hidden power and natural balance of the government "...which would be lost if it were defined." A Prince, who could so easily forgive his people when they had been in the wrong, "... cannot fail to hear them when they are in the right." While defining the ruler as the state, Aristotle also believes that the state and the individual naturally pursue the same good, although the " good," found in the state (or ruling power), is greater and nobler than the good pursued by individuals. For the Trimmer, this natural "good" rests within the natural "power" of the monarch, providing an equilibrium between liberty and law. " The crown hath power sufficient to protect our liberties. The people have so much liberty as is necessary to make them useful to the crown."

Aristotle's ideal man is very much like the Trimmer. " He is open in his dislikes and preferences; he talks and acts frankly, because of his contempt for men and things...He cannot live in complaisance with others, except it be a friend...He is not prone to vehemence, for he thinks nothing is important." Likewise, the Trimmer asserts that he cannot be bullied into agreeing with the opinions of his enemies as he "...is very much confirmed in his own (opinion) by them." Following the Aristotelian definition of the ideal man, the Trimmer declares that " ... he thinketh himself in the right, grounding his opinion upon that truth, which equally hateth to be under the oppression of wrangling Sophistry on the one hand, or the short dictates of mistaken authority on the other."

Clearly, there is no denying the political influence of Aristotle on the political writings of Halifax, especially in *The Character of a Trimmer*. The Aristotelian doctrine of the mean and the belief in the natural authority of the ruling class forms the basis for Halifax's political propositions. Halifax blatantly confirms Aristotle's affirmation that laws exist to control man's baser instincts, going so far as to borrow Aristotle's term and idea of the " beast " in man. Both political theorists are in conspicuously strong agreement concerning the inviolable bond between ruler and ruled, and both exhibit the same Machiavelian attitude towards retention of power within their generally concuring, balanced construction of goverment, that of a constitutional monarchy.

Cited From:

Aristotle, <u>Politics.</u> Ed. J.A. Smith and W.D. Ross. Oxford. 1254, a 23-4Aristotle, <u>Politics.</u> Ed. J.A. Smith and W.D. Ross. Oxford. 1254, a 23-4

Saville, George, First Marquess of Halifax. *The Complete Works of George Saville, First Marquess of Halifax*. Ed.Walter Raleigh. Oxford: Clarendon Press, 1912.

4.b. Satire On Christianity

By Mandeville [1670-1733]

In the eighteenth century, Bernard Mandeville, a Whig and an immigrant Dutchman, was regarded as a proponent of vice and an opponent of virtue and religion. Virtue and an over-zealous public spirit were ideals derided by Mandeville.

My Commentary on *Free Thoughts on Religion*

At the beginning of his full-length work on religion, *Free Thoughts on Religion*, the Church and National Happiness, Mandeville defines religion as an "acknowledgement of an immortal power." He later says that " Men of sense, and good logicians " have wasted their time arguing about the subject of religion and God, for knowledge of God is something " which no language can give them the least idea of."

Mandeville ruled out the possibilities of a rational or systematic religion, as religion was based on human comprehension, so therefore, nothing can be known about God and nothing worthwhile can be said about the subject. In *Free Thoughts*, Mandeville concentrates on a threefold critique: religious phenomena as an aspect of human behavior, an expose of the corrupt practices of the clergy through the ages, and a plea for toleration if not permissiveness.

Mandeville states in his Preface to *Free Thoughts* that it is " only bigots and the enemies of truth who would insinuate that Free Thoughts must be impious and atheistical, in the same manner as lewd debauchees by the words good natured lady would have you understand a whore."

In *Free Thoughts*, Mandeville states that men have wasted their time trying to grapple with such problems as the mystery of the holy trinity of God, on the complex idea of free will, and on predestination. Their insistence upon maintaining dogmatic positions on these religious opinions has led to violent conflict.

In Mandevill'e *An Inquiry into the Origin of Honour, and the Usefulness of Christianity in War*, Mandeville's anti-clericalism manifests itself in the expose of the vicious practices of the clergy, particularly those members of the Roman Catholic Church. "No set of people have so artfully played upon mankind as the church of Rome. In the use they made of scripture, they have consulted all of our frailties...," accusing the Christian church of exploiting human frailty for their own selfish and greedy benefit. Mandeville goes on to say that the original spirit of Christianity, simple and unaffected, was deliberately set aside and replaced by the pomp of Popery.

In *Free Thoughts* instead of Christianity being practiced at home, Christianity was practiced in magnificent churches, for he states that the clergy realized

"There is a kind of magick in a fine church. They look upon it as a rampart against hell and the Devil." Later, in *Free Thoughts*, Mandeville turns from the political aspect of religion and the control of the clergy (who set themselves up as interpreters of matters beyond human comprehension) to analyzing religious behavior in psychological terms. He considers the reasons that induce men to accept ideas contrary to reason and their senses when he comments: " ....were men to be taught from the infancy that it was a mystery, that on a certain occasion two and two made seven, with an addition to be believed on pain of damnation, I am persuaded that at least seven in ten would swallow the shameful paradox."

Mysteries are therefore accepted because people have been taught to accept these mysteries from childhood. The fact that they contradict reason is insufficient grounds for rejection. Mandeville also directs his attention to the concrete symbols and rites of the church that the clergy used to assuage mankind's need for re-assurance. In the Christian church, the most important symbol is the cross. Mandeville considers that when the cross is used excessively, this symbol is made into an object of superstition. Mandeville further explores that objects, such as priestly garments and incense, are designed to inspire awe and a sense of solemnity and holiness which particularly impresses the feeble-minded. Mandeville states cynically, that priests' robes are no "more holy or more necessary that the gowns of judges, the swordbearer's cap of maintenance or the habits of the Yeomen of the Guards."

Mandeville criticizes the unreasonableness of the mysteries of faith, as they are accepted instinctively rather than on intellectual grounds. The only explanation for these mysteries is scriptural, as they cannot be measured by the standards of reason. "Experience teaches us that this opinion (i.e. the acceptance of mysteries) is much influenced by the fears, wishes, inclinations and varies according to the capacity of the believer." Mandeville maintains that all religious instinct, including the Christian one, is based on the fear people have of death, and the fear they have of the unknown.

In *Free Thoughts*, Anglicans and dissenters argue about the non-essentials of religion:

" A churchman receives the sacrament kneeling, a Presbyterian sitting...What barbarous notions must a man have of the deity, who could imagine that, if both spoke sincerely, and otherwise took the sacrament conscientiously, tho' in different postures, God would be offended at either." It is high time, he adds, that Christians should "distinguish between the spirit of God, and that of contradiction."

Commentary on *The Fable Of The Bees*

The *Fable of the Bees* attacks self-discipline and temperance. Mandeville defends undisciplined activity. Luxury, according to the poem, " ...employed a million of the poor." In Mandeville's account, human appetites are indefinite and new wants can be invented.

In *Fable of the Bees*, vol. I, in " An Essay on Charity and Charity Schools," he states:

" As to religion, the most knowing and polite part of a nation have everywhere where the least of it; craft has a greater hand in making rogues than stupidity and vice in general is where more predominate than where arts and sciences flourish..." Mandeville further criticized the education of those who attend charity schools as being futile, as they will have little use for their education in their adult employment, as they will always be relegated to the station in life as lower class people.

In his *Origin of Honour* in Fable I, Mandeville satirizes the inconsistency which enables people to claim to be Christians, while at the same time insisting as their role as "men of honour" regulated by a military code. Christianity and the idea of warfare should be opposed. Mandeville, however, states that politicians and their clerical allies encourage unchristian notions of honor and military glory in the name of national interest and the public good.

An amusing expression of Mandeville's anti-clericalism is in his parable of the " small beer " in Fable I. The clergy allows that "small beer" may be drunk so long as men do it only to "mend their complexions." If they do it for pleasure, they indulge in vice which cannot in anyway be condoned.

In the "Grumbling Hive," Mandeville seeks to expose those bees (the hypocrites) who enjoy the (material) benefits of worldly greatness while deploring the absence of simple, virtuous living. Mandeville makes a contribution to the important 18th century debate about the relationship between material progress and moral decline. In the poem, " The Grumbling Hive," he shows the ruin that follows when Jove answers the Bees, in Horatian Manner, in their request for a return to the simple life. The moral is that "Bare virtue can't make nations live in splendor." The poem in Fable I is an attack on those hypocrites whom he sees enjoying the fruits of a prospering society while at the same time pleading their commitment to a simple, aesthetic ideal. No doubt Mandeville did regard some Christian values as desirable, but realistically as too hard for unregenerate people to achieve. Mandeville believes that real virtue is incompatible with national power and prosperity. He also considers that what the clergy calls virtue is a sham, and a cloak for their avarice and thirst for power.

In his Preface to Part I of the Fable, Mandeville states: "...to expose the unreasonableness and folly of those, that desirous of being an opulent and flourishing people, and wonderfully greedy after all the benefits they receive as such, are yet always murmuring at and exclaiming against those vices and inconveniences that from the beginning of the world to this present day, have been inseparable from all kingdoms and states that ever were fam'd for strength, riches and politeness at the same time. It is inconsistent for a state to be opulent and virtuous at the same time."

There seems to be a good deal to support Mandeville's claim that the *Fable of the Bees* "is a book of severe and exalted morality." Mandeville appears as an uncompromising ascetic, disgusted by the materialism, the selfishness, the lust, and the vanity of mankind, detecting the wickedness in the hearts of even the respectable and apparently upright, horrified at the worldliness and hypocrisy of institutionalized religion, and preaches spiritual regeneration as the only possible remedy.

In the *Fable of the Bees*, vice is an action that gratifies appetite, actions that might in some way injure society or render the actor "less serviceable to others." Virtue must go counter to nature and seek the benefit of others by conquering the passions out of a rational ambition of being good. The conversion of private vices into public benefit might incline one to celebrate with various economists the beneficial economic outcome of that depravity on world prosperity.

The Fables most explicitly attack temperance or self-discipline. Undisciplined, disproportionate activity is accepted by Mandeville, as luxury employs "a million of the poor." By Mandeville's account, human appetites are generally unbounded, and new human wants can always be invented. It is not necessary that men should simply quantitatively increase their indulgence in food, drink and sex; they will find ways of developing niceties of dress, equipage and behavior. Pride "... encourages everybody, who is conscious of his little merit, if he is any ways able, to wear clothes above his rank."

4.c. Jonathan Swift

My Commentary on Swift's Scatology: Neurosis or Rabelaisian Influence

Much has been written about Swift's preoccupation with scatology. Many critics seem to be offended by Swift's spending so much time rolling around in excrement. The post World War II, psychoanalytic Freudians have analyzed Swift's preoccupation with anality as deriving from some type of psychological disturbance which, they conjecture, Swift experienced in his childhood. In 1942, the *Psychoanalytic Review* published the following observation on Swift's mental problems, explaining that *Gulliver's Travels* presents "...abundant evidence of the neurotic makeup of the author and discloses in him a number of perverse trends indicative of fixation at the anal sadistic state of libidinal development. Most conspicuous among those perverse trends is that of coprophilia, although the work furnishes evidence of numerous other related neurotic characteristics accompanying the general picture of psychosexual infantilism and emotional immaturity" (Greenberg 275).[1]

Other critics have traced the influence of Rabelais' carnivalesque imagery on Swift's writings, especially his allusions to the functions of the lower bodily stratum such as urination and defecation. Ronald Paulson notes the similarity between Rabelais' and Swift's usage of feces as an element in satire: "...why is it a general characteristic of satire to emphasize excretion-whether as a mode of vituperation or as simply a diminishing device? This is particularly blatant in Rabelais, from whom it might be thought Swift inherits much of his concern with the excremental" (Paulson 121).

Norman O. Brown suggests that "...if we are willing to listen to Swift we will find startling anticipations of Freudian theorems about anality, about sublimation, and about the universal neurosis of mankind" (Brown 38). According to Freud, the anal stage is the second stage in the development of the sexual instinct, the first being the oral stage, and the final stage reached when the genital zone occupies the prime position of the child's attention. The anal stage, as part of the development of the child's sexual instinct, includes those bodily processes such as eating, sucking, urination, and defecation that satisfy the child's sexual instinct and infuse the child with sexual energy. Freud considers sexual perversion of adults as a phenomenon of retarded normal development, a regression to one of the three earlier stages of infantile sexuality, which should be completed by the time a child reaches the age of four or five. Freudian critics are then concerned with the question of whether Swift's preoccupation with the anal was a result of a trauma experienced during his childhood. In contrast to a Freudian analysis of Swift, the probable influence of Rabelais' methodology on Swift's writings was

---

1   Cited by Louis Landa in "Jonathan Swift," in the Norton Critical Edition of "Gulliver's Travels," ed. Robert Greenberg (New York: W.W. Norton & Co., 1961), p. 275.

first noted when Pope referred to Swift as sitting in 'Rabelais' easy chair.'[2] I have already noted that Ronald Paulson suggests that Swift's preoccupation with anality was inherited from Rabelais.

While Paulson connects excretory images in Swift's writings as part of the elements of satire, I think it is also important to focus on Mikhail Bakhtin's study on the nature of grotesque satire, which consists of improper or indecent exaggeration of the body. The image of Lemuel Gulliver's gigantic penis stuck out and peeing over the fire that threatens the Queen of Lilliput's palace is exaggerated and improper. When Gulliver acts as a human archway, through which Lilliput's troops pass under in parade, the troops are amazed at the size of his private member peeking through a hole in the crotch of his pants. The realm of the grotesque, according to Bakhtin, exaggerates the inappropriate uses of the human body, as well as indecent displays of human genitalia. Gulliver's posing as a human archway recalls Rabelais' imagery when Panurge proposed to build the walls of Paris with human genitals:

> " I have observed that the pleasure twats of women in this part of the world are much cheaper than stones. Therefore, the walls should be built of twats, symmetrically and according to the rules of architecture, the largest to go in front...What devil could possibly overthrow these walls...What is more, no lightening could strike them. Why? Because they are consecrated." (Book 2, Chapter 15)

Just as the trampiness of the Parisian women is satirized by Panurge's grotesque, indecent imagery which transforms twats to bulwarks, the lewd, sexual aggressiveness of the Brobdingnagian women is mocked through Gulliver's description of the grotesque nature of their bodies, as they attempt to sexually molest him:

> " They would often strip me naked from top to toe, and lay me at full length in their bosoms; wherewith I was much disgusted; because, to say the truth, a very offensive smell came from their skins...Their skins appeared so coarse and uneven, so variously coloured, when I saw them near, with a mole here and there as broad as a trencher...Neither did they at all scruple while I was by to discharge what they had drunk." (Chapter II, 122)

In grotesque imagery, the object of mockery is a specific negative phenomenon, something that should not exist, something that does not really exist. What should not exist in Rabelais' world is a defensive wall made of female twats, and what should not exist in Swift's world are giant, male-molesting women whose smell and skin are as offensive as their behavior. As Bakhtin sees the Rabelaisian grotesque as exaggerating and caricaturing what should not normally exist in the ordinary world, we are reminded of Gulliver's further description of

---

2   Read Alexander Pope, *The Dunciad* (London, 1729), Book I, v.20.

his sexual molestation by one of the women of Brobdingnag, who "...would set me astride upon one of her nipples, with many other tricks, wherein the reader will excuse me for not being over particular." (Chapter II, 123)

As exaggeration in the grotesque acquires an extreme fantastic character, the very nature of Gulliver's experiences in Lilliput and Brobdingnag are clear examples of the Rabelaisian tradition. What both Rabelais and Swift do satirize here, through their usage of grotesque imagery, is the inappropriate behavior of lewd women. This is not a misogynistic move on either Rabelais or Swift's part, but a mocking commentary on observed social behaviors.

Besides inappropriate exaggeration of body parts, the main elements of Rabelaisian grotesque or carnivalesque imagery include defecation, urination and swallowing, a preoccupation with the lower bodily stratum. If Swift was cognizant of these elements, he quite simply could have used this type of imagery to emphasize what he thought to be inappropriate about his society. Naturally, the Freudians disagree with such a thesis. Freud claims that the anal stage of development leads to specific character traits in adulthood such as frugality or greed. The child develops an anal eroticism by holding back feces and prolonging the excretory act. This can later be manifested in the adult who has repressed his anal eroticism in the form of hoarding material things that bear a resemblance to feces.

In a more linguistically complex move, yet associated to the above discussion, Voloshinov asserts that the verbal domain of humans include serious conflicts between inner speech and outward speech, which parallel Freud's conflicts between the conscious and the unconscious. An assumption could made then, by the Freudians, that Swift's preoccupation with verbalizing images of the anus might be derived from some sexual conflict he possessed in his unconscious. In *Do What You Will*, Aldous Huxley observes that Swift's insane hatred of the bowels is at the core of his misanthropy, as well being the prime factor for his cold relations to Stella and Vanessa. While these psychoanalytic theories may have some validity, it is impossible for anyone to know explicitly whether Swift did indeed suffer from some type of sexual dysfunctionality.

If any of Swift's writings is representative of his preoccupation with anality, it is in the description of the Yahoos. Norman Brown agrees with the theory of the development of the anal infantile stage of sexuality, for he states that "it is quite obvious that the excremental vision of the Yahoo is substantially identical with the psychoanalytical doctrine of the extensive role of anal eroticism in the formation of human culture" (Brown 43). Brown, however, commends Swift's analytic skills rather than castigating him as anally insane, as he believes that Swift was ahead of Freud in observing the connection between anal obsession and human aggression, as the Yahoos behavior manifests itself primarily in "excremental aggression."

In *The Irony of Swift*, F.R. Leavis concentrates his study on the emotional intensity of Swift's genius which confronts the reader in the Yahoos. In opposition to Brown's assertions, Leavis states that Swift's irony "...is essentially a matter of surprise and negation; its function is to defeat habit, to intimidate, and to demoralize" (Leavis 18). Leavis asserts that Swift created the Yahoos as a game of savage exhibition because it was "the insolent pleasure of the author" to do so, and that the basis of this pleasure was a demonstration of superiority, Swift's delight in having power over others. What Leavis does not perceive in Swift's alleged ego trip is the truly Freudian claim that any repression of sexual instincts, which Swift might have suffered from, could be manifested in his aggressive symbolic imagery, such as the Yahoos. As sexual repression issues from the ego, and as ego accommodates a region of the unconscious, Swift's unconscious manifests itself in what is lower, darker or immoral, perhaps representing some trauma in his infantile development from which he never recovered. For Leavis to claim that Swift's excretory imagery is intimidating and demoralizing shows a rather startling intellectual delicacy on this critic's part. I can only imagine Leavis' reaction to Hogarth's prints. Is Swift insolent? Hardly!

I prefer to approach the Yahoos from the way Bakhtin writes about the images of bodily eliminations: " Dung and urine lend a bodily character to matter, to the world, to the cosmic elements, which become closer, more intimate, more easily grasped, for this is the matter, the elemental force, born from the body itself. It transforms cosmic terror into a gay carnival monster" (Bakhtin 308). In the land of the Houynhhnms, the excrement of the Yahoos dropping from the trees become a carnival image, for it turns the utter disgust and filthiness of these humanly formed creatures into images which cannot possibly be real - this is not the way real human beings act. Humans do not throw their excrement at other people while sitting in trees.

The images of eating, defecation and urination are common to both Rabelais and Swift. Just as Pantagruel in the cradle devoured the milk of 4600 cows, the description of Gulliver's meals in Lilliput are similar in their gigantic proportions: "I took up twenty waiters in my hand, and placed them on the table; an hundred more attended below on the ground, some with dishes of meat, and some with barrells of wine...a barrel of their liquor (was) a reasonable draught." (Chapter I, 76) The banquet images in *Gulliver's Travels* - eating, drinking, and swallowing - are also closely linked to Rabelais' use of popular festival forms. The gigantic sausages which were carried in carnival processions during the Renaissance become important factors within Rabelais' writing, and his obvious influence on Swift. Bakhtin writes that "There is a significant aspect of the banquet images...This is the special relation of food to death and to the underworld. The word 'to die' had among its various connotations the meaning of 'being swallowed' or being 'eaten up.' The image of the underworld in Rabelais was also meant by him as the topographical lower bodily stratum, that which represented hell in carnival forms" (Bakhtin 301). In each of Gulliver's sojourns in Lilliput and in Brobdingnag, the imagery of food is associated with the possibility of Gulliver's death. Especially in

Brobdingnag, there is always the danger of Gulliver being eaten by a gargantuan form, as Gulliver almost becomes food himself for a monkey, a frog and a cat. Surely, in both of these places, Gulliver exists in a living hell. Rabelais' possible influence on Swift's imagery is clearly within the tradition of the popular festival imagery of the Renaissance.

When Pantagruel and his friends made preparation for battle against King Anarchus, "Pantagruel felt an imperious need of draining his bladder. So he voided their camp so freely and torrentially as to drown them all and flood the countryside ten leagues round." (Book 2, Chapter 28) The influence of this story by Rabelais is unabashedly repeated by Swift in Chapter I of *Gulliver's Travels* when Lemuel extinguishes the palace fire: " The heat I had contracted by coming very near the flames, and by my labouring to quench them, made the wine begin to be operated by urine; which I voided in such quantity...that in three minutes the fire was wholly extinguished." (Swift 68-69) While the situational motives for Pentagruel's and Gulliver's urinary eliminations differ, the very image of these giants emptying their cosmically large bladders are distinctly similar.

During the early 1730s Swift wrote a number of unprintable poems which dealt with excretory matter, such as "The Lady's Dressing Room"(1730), "Strephon and Chloe" (1731), "A Beautiful Young Nymph Going to bed" (1731), and "Cassinus and Peter" (1731). Dr. Brown singles out these poems as scandalous examples of the fact that "In his analysis of human nature there is emphasis on, and attitude toward, the anal function that is unique in Western literature" (Brown 31). In the first of these poems Celia "shits"; in the second one Chloe, in her wedding bed, has to reach for the chamber pot in order to "piss." David Nokes asserts that these poems "have done more to blacken Swift's reputation with later generations than anything else he wrote" (Nokes 365).

An example of one such poem, "Beautiful Young Nymph," is as follows:

Corinna, Pride of Drury Lane,
For whom no Shepherd sighs in vain;
Never did Covent Garden Boast
So bright a batter'd, strolling Toast;
No drunken rake to pick her up,
No cellar where on Tick to sup;
Returning at the midnight hour;
Four stories climbing to her bower;
Then seated on a three-legged Chair,
Takes off her artificial Hair:
Now, Picking out a Crystal Eye,
She wipes it clean, and lays it by.
Her Eye-Brows from a Mouse's Hyde,

Stuck on with Art on either side,

(she) Pulls out the rags contriv'd to prop
Her flabby dugs, and down they drop
Up goes her Hand, and off she slips
The Bolsters, that supply her hips.
With gentlest Touch, she next explores
Her chancres, Issues, running sores.

The poems ends with a warning to the readers that "Who sees will spew; who smells be poisoned." Swift has no pity for this prostitute, and he wants the reader to see her for the dreadful woman that she is. At the same time, Swift's preoccupation with the darker aspects of life and the human body indicate not so much a sexual obsession with women, as Swift constructs the female body as grotesque, depraved and diseased, but a preoccupation with social commentary. Swift boldly criticizes the prostitutes of his era without apology.

In "Cassinus and Peter," Swift mocks the idea of romantic love, as well as the functions of the lower bodily stratum. The poem centers on two college students at Cambridge University. Throughout the poem Peter asks Cassinus a series of questions as to why Cassinus is so depressed over his girlfriend Celia: " Is Celia dead...has she played the whore?.Has the small or greater pox/Sunk down her nose, or seamed her face?" At the end of the poem, the reader discovers that Cassinus is in such a depressive swoon because he discovered "Celia's foul disgrace...Nor wonder how I lost my wits;/ Oh! Celia, Celia, Celia shits!" Norman Brown defends Swift against Murry's charges that Swift hates women because they evacuate. Brown pursues a more universal application to the poem's theme, which is "the conflict between our animal body, appropriately epitomized in the anal function, and our pretentious sublimations, more specifically the pretensions of sublimated or romantic-Platonic love" (Brown 39).

Swift's concern with anal filth continues past his poetry into *Gulliver's Travels*. According to a number of critics such as Brown and Nokes, Swift's persistent concern with the anal might be explained by the loss of his parents in his infancy. Brown writes about this loss that, "Swift lost his father before he was born; was kidnapped from his mother only three years later, only to be abandoned by his mother one month after his return to her at the psychoanalytically crucial Oedipal period. By psychoanalytical standards such a succession of infantile traumata must establish more than a predisposition to life long neurosis" (Brown 35) According to Freud, the most important event in a child's subconscious is his sexual attraction to his mother and his hatred for his father. " The libido continues time and time again to be impelled toward the mother, sexualizing all her attentions and services; the activities of being nursed, being bathed, being helped with defecation, and so forth" (Voloshinov 32). All of a man's future love relations become only a surrogate for his first love, a love that had been bonded by the child's complete organic unity with its mother. It could logically follow that Swift's abandonment by his mother would have irrevocably damaged his unconscious, evidenced by his preoccupation with anality and defecation, the second stage of infantile sexual development. The question becomes whether Swift actually suffered from an arrested sexual development at the second stage of his sexual development causing his scatological preoccupations. The problem with this type of psychoanalytic criticism of Swift is that the Freudians base their criticism on what was hidden within Swift's unconscious, conjecturing about his relationship with his mother, female friends etc.. This type of autobiographical analysis is impossible to be proven to be true or to be accurate.

Fortunately, Norman Brown defends Swift against the charges of insanity, which had been issued by Huxley who thought "Swift is the excremental vision," and by Murry and other psychoanalysts. Brown believes that "Psychoanalysis ...is necessary in order to sustain the requisite posture of humility-about ourselves, about mankind, and towards genius. It is also necessary in order to take seriously the Swiftian exploration of the universal exploration of mankind" (Brown 38). While Huxley charges Swift with insanity, rather than dealing with Swift's characterization of Gulliver's madness, Bakhtin explains that the theme of madness is also inherent to all grotesque forms, because madness is a "... gay parody of official reason, of the narrow seriousness of official truth." When Gulliver returns to England at the end of his travels, he has lost his sanity. He views the human form as representative of the Yahoo, and is even repelled by the smell of his wife. Gulliver's madness is evident when he says: " My horses understood me tolerably well; I converse with them at least four hours every day...they live in great amity with me, and friendship to each other" (Swift.272). Gulliver's eventual madness is a gay parody of the official reason of the Houyhnhnms rational horses, which quite possibly could be a parody on Swift's own notions of officialdom. I cannot help but think that Swift might be admitting to his personal madness with regards his affiliation to the Anglican church.

If we discuss the appropriateness of Swift's scatology in relation to Christianity, then "...excrement is both a natural symbol of the defilement of the soul by sin, and a reminder of the punishment of mortality for Adam's original sin since excretory functions are part of the digestive process and can symbolize change and mutability" (Frontain 301). As a Christian satirist, Swift could quite consciously emphasize the nastiest aspects of the body in order to uncover what people like to disguise, namely their vices. As vices are usually manifested within the lower bodily stratum, it is possible that Swift found this type of imagery appropriate to his moral message. In "The Comedy of Swift's Scatological Poetry," Thomas Gilmore attempts to summarize the views of critics who view Swift as a moral messenger: " Generally they concur that Swift here is the Christian preacher and satiric moralist seeking to humble man's pride by satirizing fornication. Specifically, they also agree, Swift seeks to explode man's illusions about romantic love by revealing the body at its filthiest" (Gilmore 33). Swift even treated religious enthusiasm as something that was the product of the lower material bodily stratum, when he wrote that religiosity was "the Product of Natural Causes, the effect of Strong Imagination, Spleen, violent anger, Fear, Grief, Pain, and the like." Norman Brown links Swift's sublimated anality to religious preaching, as in *A Tale of a Tub* when the preachers reach orgasmic heights by shiting in barrels. And finally, Bakhtin believes that images of urine and dung as cosmic bodily matter merely defeat whatever cosmic fears institutions like religion impose on man.

While Freudian theories of Swift's scatology have some merit, Swift's preoccupation with anality could simply be derived from his century's literary traditions. Swift could have been caught up in bawdiness because bawdiness was what his era was all about. Whether or not Swift purposely copied Rabelaisian imagery can never be positively proven, although Swift's inheriting the Renaissance traditions of grotesque imagery seems a more plausible and logical explanation for Swift's usage of fecal imagery than does his inheriting a problematic fecal subconscious. Irvin Ehrenpreis makes an enlightened comment on Swift's usage of obscenity: "Swift's writings is sometimes coarse or bawdy...If we are shocked, let us admit it is traditions that shock us, not the man" (Ehrenpreis 49). Ehrenpreis emphasizes that what we might call obscene today was not thought to be so by Swift's contemporaries. Or, could it be, perhaps, that Swift was quite simply having a hell of a rollicking good time?

Works Cited

Bakhtin, Mikhail *Rabelais and His World*, trans. Helene Iswolsky. Bloomington: Indiana University Press, 1984.

Brown, Norman O. "The Excremental vision," *Life Against Death: The Psychoanalytical Meaning of History*. Middletown.:Wesleyan University Press, 1959.

Ehrenpreis, Irvin. *The Personality of Swift*. London: Methuen & Company, 1958.

Frontain, Raymond-Jean. "Scatology in Swift's Satire," *Critical Approaches to Teaching Swift*. New York: AMS Press, 1992.

Gilmore,Thomas B. " The Comedy of Swift's Scatological Poetry," *PMLA* 91 (1976), p.33.

Greenberg, Robert, ed. "Jonathan Swift," in the *Norton Critical Edition of "Gulliver's Travels* .New York: W.W. Norton & Co., 1961.

Leavis, F.R. "The Irony of Swift." *A Collection of Critical Essays*. Ed. Ernest Tuveson. New Jersey: Prentice Hall, 1964.

Nokes, David. *Jonathan Swift,A Hypocrite Reversed:A Critical Biography*. Oxford: Oxford University Press, 1985.

Paulson, Ronald. *Theme and Structure in Swift's Tale of a Tub*. New Haven: Yale University Press, 1960.

Pope, Alexander. *The Dunciad*. London, 1729, Book I, v.20.

Voloshinov, V.N. *Freudianism:A Critical Sketch*. Bloomington and Indianapolis: Indiana University Press, 1976..

Section

S ection | V

Reading Religion

5.a. Zecharia Sitchin

I have spent the majority of my life reading and studying about varied religions—too many to add to this book. One author who has made a profound impact on my recent thinking is Dr. Zecharia Sitchin. Sitchin was born in Russia, raised in Palestine, and graduated from the University of London with a degree in economic history. He worked for years as a journalist and editor in Israel before settling in New York. Sitchin believes <u>ancient visitors from other worlds</u> came to earth and created the first man. His key ideas assume that ancient myths are not myths but historical and scientific texts. According to Sitchin, ancient Sumerian clay tablets reveal that gods from another planet (Nibiru, which orbits our Sun every 3,600 years) arrived on Earth some 450,000 years ago and created humans by <u>genetic engineering</u>. I suggest you get the

Earth Chronicle *series—my favorite book of the Chronicles is* Divine Encounters. *I do not ascribe to all of Sitchin's theories, but find his scholarship of the ancient world very entertaining.*

The Case of Adam's Alien Genes
by Zecharia Sitchin

Thinking About Human Origins: Writing Religion

- **Human beings have a collective unconsciousness about their true origins.** Research Zecharia Sitchin's theories about the origins of the human race in <u>The Earth Chronicles.</u>

- How would his theories topple existing religious establishments?

- Would his theories unite or further divide the world?

- I would like you to research the ancient gods of Sumer. Find out their names and where they came from. Research the language of the Bible to find connections with these people. Start by reading anything by or about Dr. Zecharia Sitchin. Construct a grid to organize your research; for example,

Names of Gods	Origin/ Geneaology	Family Relations	Off- spring	Other Names Used	Region on Earth Ruled	Space-port Locations	Etc.
Anu							
Enki							
Enlil							
Ninshur'hag (many spelling variations)							
Etc.							

- You can expand the grid with other information categories—as many as you like. After you have collected this information, try to find similarities/connections among the categories; discuss your findings in an analytic way. This must be a substantial discussion.

In whose image was The Adam – the prototype of modern humans, Homo sapiens – created? The Bible asserts that the *Elohim* said: "Let us fashion the Adam in our image and after our likeness." But if one is to accept a tentative explanation for enigmatic genes that humans possess, offered when the deciphering of the human genome was announced in mid-February, the feat was decided upon by a group of bacteria!

"Humbling" was the prevalent adjective used by the scientific teams and the media to describe the principal finding – that the human genome contains not the anticipated 100,000 - 140,000 genes (the stretches of DNA that direct the production of amino-acids and proteins) but only some 30,000+ — little more than double the 13,601 genes of a fruit fly and barely fifty percent more than the roundworm's 19,098. What a comedown from the pinnacle of the genomic Tree of Life!

Moreover, there was hardly any uniqueness to the human genes. They are comparative to not the presumed 95 percent but to almost 99 percent of the chimpanzees, and 70 percent of the mouse. Human genes, with the same functions, were found to be identical to genes of other vertebrates, as well as invertebrates, plants, fungi, even yeast. The findings not only confirmed that there was one source of DNA for all life on Earth, but also enabled the scientists to trace the evolutionary process – how more complex organisms evolved, genetically, from simpler ones, adopting at each stage the genes of a lower life form to create a more complex higher life form – culminating with Homo sapiens.

The "Head-scratching" Discovery

It was here, in tracing the vertical evolutionary record contained in the human and the other analyzed genomes, that the scientists ran into an enigma. The "head-scratching discovery by the public consortium," as <u>Science</u> termed it, was that the human genome contains 223 genes that do not have the required predecessors on the genomic evolutionary tree.

How did Man acquire such a bunch of enigmatic genes?

In the evolutionary progression from bacteria to invertebrates (such as the lineages of yeast, worms, flies or mustard weed – which have been deciphered) to vertebrates (mice, chimpanzees) and finally modern humans, these 223 genes are completely missing in the invertebrate phase. Therefore, the scientists can explain their presence in the human genome by a "rather recent" (in evolutionary time scales) "probable horizontal transfer from bacteria."

In other words: At a relatively recent time as Evolution goes, modern humans acquired an extra 223 genes not through gradual evolution, not vertically on the Tree of Life, but horizontally, as a sideways insertion of genetic material from bacteria...

An Immense Difference

Now, at first glance it would seem that 223 genes is no big deal. In fact, while every single gene makes a great difference to every individual, 223 genes make an immense difference to a species such as ours.

The human genome is made up of about three billion neucleotides (the "letters" A-C-G-T which stand for the initials of the four nucleic acids that spell out all life on Earth); of them, just a little more than one percent are grouped into functioning genes (each gene consists of thousands of "letters"). The difference between one individual person and another amounts to about one "letter" in a thousand in the DNA "alphabet." The difference between Man and Chimpanzee is less than one percent as genes go; and one percent of 30,000 genes is 300. So, 223 genes is more than two thirds of the difference between me, you and a chimpanzee!

An analysis of the functions of these genes through the proteins that they spell out, conducted by the Public Consortium team and published in the journal <u>Nature</u>, shows that they include not only proteins involved in important physiological but also psychiatric functions. Moreover, they are responsible for important neurological enzymes that stem only from the mitochondrial portion of the DNA – the so-called "Eve" DNA that humankind inherited only through the mother-line, all the way back to a single "Eve." That finding alone raises doubt regarding that the "bacterial insertion" explanation.

A Shaky Theory

How sure are the scientists that such important and complex genes, such an immense human advantage, was obtained by us —"rather recently"— through the courtesy of infecting bacteria? "It is a jump that does not follow current evolutionary theories," said Steven Scherer, director of mapping of the Human Genome Sequencing Center, Baylor College of Medicine.

"We did not identify a strongly preferred bacterial source for the putative horizontally transferred genes," states the report in <u>Nature</u>. The Public Consortium team, conducting a detailed search, found that some 113 genes (out of the 223) "are widespread among bacteria" – though they are entirely absent even in invertebrates. An analysis of the proteins which the enigmatic genes express showed that out of 35 identified, only ten had counterparts in vertebrates (ranging from cows to rodents to fish); 25 of the 35 were unique to humans.

"It is not clear whether the transfer was from bacteria to human or from human to bacteria," <u>Science</u> quoted Robert Waterson, co-director of Washington University's Genome Sequencing Center, as saying.

But if Man gave those genes to bacteria, where did Man acquire those genes to begin with?

The Role of the Anunnaki

Readers of my books must be smiling by now, for they know the answer.

They know that the biblical verses dealing with the fashioning of The Adam are condensed renderings of much much more detailed Sumerian and Akkadian texts, found inscribed on clay tablets, in which the role of the Elohim in Genesis is performed by the Anunnaki – "Those Who From Heaven to Earth Came."

As detailed in my books, beginning with The 12th Planet (1976) and even more so in Genesis Revisited and The Cosmic Code, the Anunnaki came to Earth some 450,000 years ago from the planet Nibiru – a member of our own solar system whose great orbit brings it to our part of the heavens once every 3,600 years. They came here in need of gold, with which to protect their dwindling atmosphere. Exhausted and in need of help in mining the gold, their chief scientist Enki suggested that they use their genetic knowledge to create the needed Primitive Workers. When the other leaders of the Anunnaki asked: How can you create a new being? He answered:

"The being that we need already exists; all that we have to do is put our mark on it."

The time was some 300,000 years ago.

What he had in mind was to upgrade genetically the existing hominids, who were already on Earth through Evolution, by adding some of the genes of the more advanced Anunnaki. That the Anunnaki, who could already travel in space 450,000 years ago, possessed the genomic science (whose threshold we have now reached) is clear not only from the actual texts but also from numerous depictions in which the double-helix of the DNA is rendered as Entwined Serpents (a symbol still used for medicine and healing) — see illustration 'A' below.

When the leaders of the Anunnaki approved the project (as echoed in the biblical "Let us fashion the Adam"), Enki with the help of Ninharsag, the Chief Medical Officer of the Anunnaki, embarked on a process of genetic engineering, by adding and combining genes of the Anunnaki with those of the already-existing hominids. When, after much trial and error breathtakingly described and recorded in antiquity, a "perfect model" was attained, Ninharsag held him up and shouted: "My hands have made it!" An ancient artist depicted the scene on a cylinder seal (illustration 'B'). And that, I suggest, is how we had come to possess the unique extra genes. It was in the image of the Anunnaki, not of bacteria, that Adam and Eve were fashioned.

A Matter of Extreme Significance

Unless further scientific research can establish, beyond any doubt, that the only possible source of the extra genes are indeed bacteria, and unless it is then also determined that the infection ("horizontal transfer") went from bacteria to Man and not from Man to bacteria, the only other available solution will be that offered by the Sumerian texts millennia ago.

Until then, the enigmatic 223 alien genes will remain as an alternative – and as a corroboration by modern science of the Anunnaki and their genetic feats on Earth.

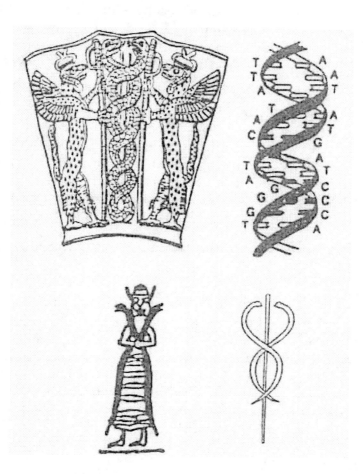

Illustration A

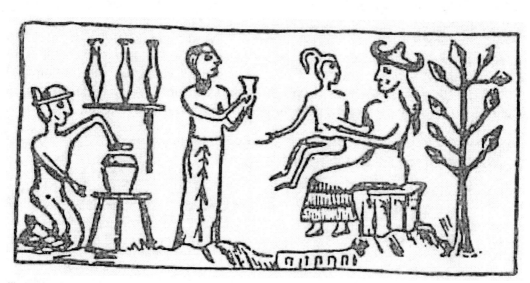

Illustration B

The report of the Public Consortium is in <u>Nature</u>, Feb 15, 2001 and of Celera
Genomics in <u>Science</u> of Feb 16th, 2001.

Will Biblical Prophecies be Fulfilled?

By Zecharia Sitchin

The War in Iraq and *The Earth Chronicles* "War has come to the cradle of civilization,
" current headlines have been announcing; and both fans and interviewers have
asked me what is my "take" on these events. "How strange that 6000 years of
human history keep leading us to devastation in this ancient place; I wonder if
you have any thoughts on this issue," asked a fan from England. "Is this the
fulfillment of biblical prophecies?" asked an interviewer.

Indeed, today's Iraq encompasses ancient Mesopotamia, the Land Between
the Rivers where Assyria and Babylon and long before them Sumer had flourished.
It is there, <u>geographically</u>, where the first known civilization had blossomed out,
giving Mankind the firsts in writing and literature, the wheel and the kiln, art and
music, mathematics and astronomy, kingship and laws, temples and religion,
and the first Cities of Man, among them the famed Ur whence Abraham had
come.

Preserving The Legacy

The issue of preserving and respecting that ancient legacy is perhaps best illustrated
by Ur's mighty ziggurat (step pyramid) whose ruins still dominate the landscape.
In the first Gulf War, the Iraqis placed their aircraft next to the ziggurat, expecting
(correctly!) that the Americans would not risk bombing the planes for fear of
damaging the ziggurat; the Iraqis did it again this time – but this time (according
to unconfirmed reports) the airfield was captured by Special Forces without a
bomb dropped.

While the Iraqis converted a symbol of Sumer's legacy into a military target, it is known that in Washington panels of archeologists and other scholars have been advising the campaign planners on the location and importance of ancient sites. It has been pointed out, however, that various dam and irrigation projects have obliterated potential archeological sites; and although in the first Gulf War war-damage was minimal, post-war looting of sites and museums was rampant

The Wars of Men

War – any war – entails carnage and destruction, and a time of No More Wars was deemed already in biblical times as the idyllic time when swords shall be made into ploughshares. Yet wars accompanied Mankind from the earliest times, and the Lands of the Bible, encompassing today's Iraq, have known war after war after war.

Today's Iraq was artificially put together by the victorious Allies after World War I, in the 1920's. Today's capital, Baghdad (which is not ancient Babylon) was established by invading Arabs in AD 750 and was overrun by Mongol hordes in AD 1469. Greeks (under Alexander the Great), Persians, Medians, Sassanians, Parthians warred there. And the great international war recorded in the Bible, of the Kings of the East against the Kings of the West, took place in the time of Abraham.

The kingdoms that followed Sumer, Babylonia and Assyria, turned war into a permanent state policy; their kings boasted in their annals of one campaign after another. Killings, annihilations, destruction, pillaging, subjugation fill the records.

In Who's Footsteps?

While ancient Sumer knew wars (its monuments indeed depict soldiers and war chariots), its kings boasted of assuring peace, and the highest epithet for a ruler was to be called a Righteous Shepherd. The present ruthless ruler of Iraq chose as his model, however, not a Sumerian king but the Babylonian Nebuchadnezzar, the one who captured Jerusalem and destroyed the Temple that Solomon built for Yahweh.

Saddam Hussein rebuilt (on a reduced scale) Babylon, not Ur or Nippur; and like the olden kings had each brick stamped with an honorific inscription – paying homage to "Saddam Hussein, protector of civilization, who rebuilt the palace, which belonged to Nebuchadnezzar."

Like that Babylonian king, Saddam Hussein spoke of Iraqi domination from the Persian Gulf (the ancient "Lower Sea") to the Mediterranean (the "Upper Sea"), of capturing Jerusalem, of destroying the "Zionist State" (alias ancient Zion).

Biblical Prophecies

By comparing Iraq to ancient Babylon and himself to Nebuchadnezzar, Saddam Hussein inescapably brings to mind the biblical prophecies concerning the kingdom that turned greatness to evil and the king whose rule brought slaughter and destruction.

The prophet Isaiah foretold the demise and destruction of Babylon by armies from a distant land, even from the skies (!) (Chapter 13) and prophesied the fate of Babylon's king and his sons (!) (Chapter 14). The prophet Jeremiah, recording the evils of Babylon and its rulers, foretold the coming punishment: "A sound of battle is in the land and a great destruction… A sword is upon the Chaldeans and upon the inhabitants of Babylon, upon her princes and upon her counselors; a sword is upon her liars… a sword is upon her mighty men." As much as the biblical prophets were for Peace, they deemed war in punishment of evil as justified.

Of First Things and Last Things

Do biblical prophecies hold true just for the time they were uttered, or are they of eternal validity, holding true for posterity whenever the circumstances are the same? Was evil punishable only then, not now? Were messianic expectations valid only B.C. and not A.D.? The question has filled volumes; I tend to agree with those who view biblical prophecies as eternally valid.

The New Testament's Book of Revelation's assertion "I am Alpha and I am Omega," I am the First and I am the Last, re-expressed the more encompassing Old Testament (or Hebrew Bible) credo of all the prophets _that The First Things Shall Be The Last Things_. Indeed, it was the knowledge of what had been that was the basis for foretelling what will be; or, as I put it in my lectures, _the Past is the Future_.

That history will repeat itself, there should be no doubt. What remains a mystery is what chapter of history will be repeated when – are we still in the middle of the what I named _The Earth Chronicles_, or is the grand cycle nearing completion and the very First Things shall fulfill the prophecies of The Return? In this regard it behooves us to recall that before the Cities of Man there had been cities of the gods and before the wars of men there were the wars of the gods –

including the one in 2024 B.C., when the use of nuclear weapons caused the demise of the Sumerian civilization.

I do recommend that my fans re-read my books, especially *The 12th Planet, The Wars of Gods and Men,* and *The Lost Book of Enki.*

April 2003
ZECHARIA SITCHIN
Reprint of this article is permitted
providing they include the copyright statement:
© Z. Sitchin 2003

5.b. ISAIAH c.777 - c.692 BC

Hebrew Prophet

As the Assyrian empire threatened the existence of Israel, the prophet Isaiah proclaimed that the threat was a warning from God to a godless people.

Isaiah urged the kings of Judah to pursue justice and avoid dangerous alliances, trusting in God's protection instead. Isaiah said that if God decides the destiny of nations, security is for God to grant and for men to deserve. Isaiah promised that a messiah would eventually appear to offer salvation.

Isaiah was witness to one of the most turbulent political and the religious periods in Jerusalem's history, and was the most "political" of the prophets. During Assyrian expansionism, he advised passive political and military approaches. Every "earthly" attempt to alter the course of events was foredoomed, since the mighty Assyria was no more than a "rod" in God's hands with which to punish the sins of Jerusalem. Isaiah took a dim view of King Hezekiah's attempts to forge alliances with Egypt and with the envoys of the Babylonian king Merodach-baladan, as a tool against Assyrian expansionism. The Christian traditions states that Isaiah, likely of aristocratic blood, was killed by being sawed in half (Hebrews 11:37).

CHAPTER 13

Thinking and Writing About Religious Language

- After reading the passage below, determine what is the most difficult part of reading scripture: is it the language? The sense of doom and gloom?

- George W. Bush's use of moral and religious rhetoric is far from unique in the American presidency; moral and religious rhetoric is a strategic tool presidents use to enhance their constitutional authority.

- How have the current candidates for the Presidency used religious language to create their moral identity for voting constituencies?

- Has the religious language become detached from policy arguments?

- Can rhetorical choices cause political effects?

- How can politicians maximize the strategic utility of moral and religious rhetoric?

- How does your personal identity make you respond to religious-political rhetoric?

- Investigate some current religious conflict—Buddhist monks in Myanmar and Tibet, Christians and Muslims in the Sudan and Nigeria, Jews and

Muslims in Israel and other countries in the Middle East etc.. **I want you explore the language used in one of the conflicts, and show how religious identity is inherent in ethnic identities and how these identities cause political conflict.**

- I would like you discuss the languages used to identify particular religions; for example, traditional Roman Catholics used to pray in Latin, and the Muslims in the Middle East pray in Arabic, etc. What other languages are used to express other religions? Do religious languages unify or create divides? Write analytically; do not just give me streams of data.

1: The oracle concerning Babylon which Isaiah the son of Amoz saw.

2: On a bare hill raise a signal, cry aloud to them; wave the hand for them to enter the gates of the nobles.

3: I myself have commanded my consecrated ones, have summoned my mighty men to execute my anger, my proudly exulting ones.

4: Hark, a tumult on the mountains as of a great multitude! Hark, an uproar of kingdoms, of nations gathering together! The LORD of hosts is mustering a host for battle.

5: They come from a distant land, from the end of the heavens, the LORD and the weapons of his indignation, to destroy the whole earth.

6: Wail, for the day of the LORD is near; as destruction from the Almighty it will come!

7: Therefore all hands will be feeble, and every man's heart will melt,

8: and they will be dismayed. Pangs and agony will seize them; they will be in anguish like a woman in travail. They will look aghast at one another; their faces will be aflame.

9: Behold, the day of the LORD comes, cruel, with wrath and fierce anger, to make the earth a desolation and to destroy its sinners from it.

10: For the stars of the heavens and their constellations will not give their light; the sun will be dark at its rising and the moon will not shed its light.

11: I will punish the world for its evil, and the wicked for their iniquity; I will put an end to the pride of the arrogant, and lay low the haughtiness of the ruthless.

12: I will make men more rare than fine gold, and mankind than the gold of Ophir.

13: Therefore I will make the heavens tremble, and the earth will be shaken out of its place, at the wrath of the LORD of hosts in the day of his fierce anger.

14: And like a hunted gazelle, or like sheep with none to gather them, every man will turn to his own people, and every man will flee to his own land.

15: Whoever is found will be thrust through, and whoever is caught will fall by the sword.

16: Their infants will be dashed in pieces before their eyes; their houses will be plundered and their wives ravished.

17: Behold, I am stirring up the Medes against them, who have no regard for silver and do not delight in gold.

18: Their bows will slaughter the young men; they will have no mercy on the fruit of the womb; their eyes will not pity children.

19: And Babylon, the glory of kingdoms, the splendor and pride of the Chalde'ans, will be like Sodom and Gomor'rah when God overthrew them.

20: It will never be inhabited or dwelt in for all generations; no Arab will pitch his tent there, no shepherds will make their flocks lie down there.

21: But wild beasts will lie down there, and its houses will be full of howling creatures; there ostriches will dwell, and there satyrs will dance.

22: Hyenas will cry in its towers, and jackals in the pleasant palaces; its time is close at hand and its days will not be prolonged.

CHAPTER 54

1: "Sing, O barren one, who did not bear; break forth into singing and cry aloud, you who have not been in travail! For the children of the desolate one will be more than the children of her that is married, says the LORD.

2: Enlarge the place of your tent, and let the curtains of your habitations be stretched out; hold not back, lengthen your cords and strengthen your stakes.

3: For you will spread abroad to the right and to the left, and your descendants will possess the nations and will people the desolate cities.

4: "Fear not, for you will not be ashamed; be not confounded, for you will not be put to shame; for you will forget the shame of your youth, and the reproach of your widowhood you will remember no more.

5: For your Maker is your husband, the LORD of hosts is his name; and the Holy One of Israel is your Redeemer, the God of the whole earth he is called.

6: For the LORD has called you like a wife forsaken and grieved in spirit, like a wife of youth when she is cast off, says your God.

7: For a brief moment I forsook you, but with great compassion I will gather you.

8:      In overflowing wrath for a moment I hid my face from you, but with everlasting love I will have compassion on you, says the LORD, your Redeemer.

9:      "For this is like the days of Noah to me: as I swore that the waters of Noah should no more go over the earth, so I have sworn that I will not be angry with you and will not rebuke you.

10:      For the mountains may depart and the hills be removed, but my steadfast love shall not depart from you, and my covenant of peace shall not be removed, says the LORD, who has compassion on you.

11:      "O afflicted one, storm-tossed, and not comforted, behold, I will set your stones in antimony, and lay your foundations with sapphires.

12:      I will make your pinnacles of agate, your gates of carbuncles, and all your wall of precious stones.

13:      All your sons shall be taught by the LORD, and great shall be the prosperity of your sons.

14:      In righteousness you shall be established; you shall be far from oppression, for you shall not fear; and from terror, for it shall not come near you.

15:      If any one stirs up strife, it is not from me; whoever stirs up strife with you shall fall because of you.

16:      Behold, I have created the smith who blows the fire of coals, and produces a weapon for its purpose. I have also created the ravager to destroy;

17:      no weapon that is fashioned against you shall prosper, and you shall confute every tongue that rises against you in judgment. This is the heritage of the servants of the LORD and their vindication from me, says the LORD."

5.c. Chapter taken from: *Letters from the Moralist*

By Dr. Deborah Coulter-Harris

LETTER: No. 19

" And they read from the book,
from the law of God, clearly,
with interpretation,
and they gave the sense,
so that the people understood the reading."

(Nehemiah 8:8)

Reading Scripture

In the attempt to process cognitively the density of prophetic literature, I want to combine my reading efforts with the equally dense theory of aesthetic response by Wolfgang Iser. Iser disagrees with the traditional method of extracting the "hidden meaning" of a text, which he considers to be "subtracted" from a literary work as a function of interpretation. Iser rebuffs the idea that meaning is a "buried secret" which reduces texts to objects which contain simple referential meaning, for, as Iser notes, "meaning cannot be reduced to a thing," such as a secret message or a hidden philosophy of life. It is for this reason, that I sometimes embrace Iser as a guide to open further gates for my travels into prophecy.

Iser explains that, as the text and the reader collectively merge into one locality, the great division between subject and object is no longer applicable; thus, meaning is no longer a definable object, but is an "effect to be experienced." As a student of literature, I was trained to engage in a type of traditional, textual analysis, where the search for this "hidden meaning" ignored the reality of the author's intentional meaning, and also overlooked any linguistic expectations that the language of the text might have proposed, which has been an obvious flaw in past biblical interpretations. Therefore, I was originally trained as an excavator of meaning, rather than as an experiencer of the effect of meaning.

The traditional interpretation of texts, which Iser describes, came from a time when literary texts were supposed to be representative of the "spirit" of their age, as well as representative of the age's social conditions, and indicative of the neuroses of the authors. Iser believes that New Criticism "called off the search for meaning," and focused on the interaction of elements within a literary work which removed the text's ambiguities, a distinctly functional approach. Iser criticizes this approach in its "attempts to define these functions through the same norms of interpretation that were used in uncovering representative meanings."[1]

---

1   Wolfgang Iser, *The Act of Reading: A Theory of Aesthetic Response* (Baltimore: The John Hopkins University Press, 1978) 15.

Iser continues to say that, "A function is not meaning - it brings about an effect, and this effect cannot be measured by the same criteria as are used in evaluating the appearance of truth."

Iser prefers to construct a method of "consistency-building" for the reader, as a structure, which guides the comprehension of the text. This structure places more emphasis on the reader of the text than on the text itself, a decidedly subjective approach, and contrary to everything biblical interpreters have been previously taught. This method of consistency, together with the continued applications of classical norms of interpretations, helps the reader to establish the consistency of "available sections of the text...which makes the unfamiliar accessible if not controllable." Iser believes that the reader's goal should not be about explaining a work, but should be about revealing the "conditions that bring about its positive effects." As a reader, I must then attempt to respond to the structure of this consistency, so that what I do not understand about the context of a piece of scripture can be controlled, as I proceed to build other aspects of the scriptural text to promote consistency in my comprehension, and as I understand how these consistencies bring me to a higher cognitive awareness of the scripture's fuller meaning.

As reading is the primary precondition for scriptural interpretation, the central focus for reading is the interaction between the prophet's text, or what Iser labels the "artistic pole," and my own reader response, or "aesthetic pole." These poles unite to create the type of meaning that Iser considers a "dynamic happening." This metaphorical socialization occurs between scripture and reader, which ascribes meaning to the phenomenon of aesthetic response and meaning making.

What I especially value about Iser is that he proposes that the experience that a reader has with a text depends on the reader's own "treasure house of experience." This subjectivity is part of the process of comprehension, where the readers' aesthetic responses restructure their experience, an experience which either "distorts or ignores" certain aspects of the reading process. Now, the experiences that I bring to the scriptural text must include my education, gender, social status, cultural affiliations and associations, supernatural experiences, and everything else that has been a factor in making me who I am as a reader, as a spiritual experiencer. If I agree with what Iser has to say, then I must restructure my own understanding of myself and my personal background, so that I do not ignore or misrepresent what the scriptural text has to say. This new awareness of personal power raises my consciousness, as I respond to scripture, so that I do not damage the meaning of scripture through my lack of understanding of the association among my "experiences," and the experience of the process of comprehension during my reading, and the experience of the prophets themselves.

Iser defines the ideal reader as someone possessing the identical, cultural codes of the author, a notion Iser believes to be quite impossible, as ideal readers would have to grasp the potential meaning of a text outside the framework of their own "historical situation." The historical qualities of a text may construct an image of an ideal reader, or help to imagine the intentions of the author, but they can never predict how the reader will respond to a particular text. As the text of scripture was meant for all generations, I believe that, as a reader, I can ignore most of the historical situation of prophecy in order to grasp higher meanings. Instead of an ideal reader, Iser believes that the role of the reader is structured by the text's varied perspectives, and by that point of convergence where the reader is able to join these perspectives, forming an interaction of perspectives. Thus, readers construct meaning by allowing this convergence of perspectives to guide them.

Thus, this "dynamic interaction" between the scriptural text and the reader becomes an event that creates a new reality. The convergence of text and reader is successful, when those conventions, common to the author and the reader, are recognized and explored. (In the case of scripture, I would assume an overpowering love of God might be one point of convergence.) These conventions are renamed by Iser as the repertoire of the text, and consist of everything which is familiar to the reader within the text, and which include allusions, understanding of social and historical context, etc.. Repertoire connects the reader to the text, as scripture becomes then for me something like a "halfway house between past and future."

The function of my use of repertoire will not only answer questions of cultural and social norms represented in scripture, but will also incorporate the traditions of written scripture that have represented these norms. Social norms and literary allusions constitute the two basic components of the repertoire, and are respectively representational of thought systems and past reactions to historical problems in scripture. As a recipient of the scriptural text, I react to my own "reality," which as I understand it, comes from my own personal storehouse of experiences, so that this reality can be reshaped and reshaped to adjust to the experience of the new repertoire, and corrects the deficiencies of both the scriptural text and my reading of it.

Iser uses "strategies" as the organizing plan for the material of the text, or for whatever references the repertoire contains. These strategies, analogous to the controlling concepts utilized in synthesis, also select those social norms of the text, which establish a frame of reference within whatever thought system or social system that the repertoire includes. Strategies then organize the perspectives of my scriptural text with my own reader's perspectives, so that comprehension is possible, while, at the same time, allowing me to recognize those perspectives initially hidden to me in other segments of scripture. Thus, I am also made aware of my own possible deficiencies in responding to scripture.

Readers are sometimes frustrated by the multiple perspectives of scriptural text. The most complicated part of reading scripture is the building of connections and consistencies. Frustration often occurs between a prophet's ancient repertoire and the personal repertoire a modern seeker/reader brings to the text. One way of building biblical consistencies is to close the gaps in the reading of scriptural text, from which we plan to derive meaning. The gaps a reader of scripture encounters are those places in the text where the reader pauses to make meaning, the place in the text where the reader lacks the information needed to cognitively process the text. When these gaps occur, the reader pauses to examine the prophet's intent, and what the prophet means through his various phrases and metaphors.

Our modern perspective of prophets' texts naturally affects our constructions of meaning; we possess acculturated perspectives, environmentally conditioned religious beliefs, and private political biases and intentions, and economic circumstances. Often, the themes we construct in response to scripture reflect our private interests, so that we frequently find a theme or construct one in our own personal reaction to the reading.

I like to build my own repertoire about what I could believe the speaker of the scripture means, and this construction is not only based upon my knowledge and academic expertise, but also upon what the Spirit has revealed, and upon what I have experienced of the supernatural. But first, I need to ask myself, what are the things I already know about the text of prophecy? How will I achieve consistency in my response to prophetic scripture, by closing the gaps between my personal repertoire and the utterances of the prophet?

The cognitive complexities of reading prophecy will rely on the level of my critical competency, on my critical literacy as a reader, and on the connections I must make between first-hand supernatural experience and the given biblical text. Within aesthetic response, the cognitive processes I engage in will come from biblical sources, and will be fashioned in response to four cognitive processing categories.

As I observe what the prophet has written, I will first attempt to comprehend, according to Iser's plan, what the prophet meant by his words. This will be my first task, that of monitoring, that is, how will I build my response to the text? I will then attempt to elaborate on the prophet's text, produce my own meaning, in order to enhance both the text of prophecy, and my own personal text which I have produced as a response to the prophet's utterances. This stage involves my own repertoire of knowledge, and my competence in operating my own cognitive processing abilities. At this phase my prior knowledge and spiritual experiences combine with the biblical text to create new propositions, ideas, and critical perspectives. This is when I make the move from reading to writing; this is the origin and creation of my written response.

Now I proceed onto the structuring phase of my cognitive response; here I must determine how to shape or reshape the material; here I manipulate new propositions in the source text to create a text of my own; here I decide what propositions I agree or disagree with, and I arrange these proposition into categories, according to their cognitive complexities. At this stage I attempt to discover relations between the various propositions in the text, and my response to them; I also construct categories which are hierarchical in terms of complexity and importance, and place them in descending subordinate positions, that is, from the cognitively complex to the cognitively less complex.

Finally, the planning or shaping stage of my written response to scripture commences, as I deal with contextual ideas in the source text, or from those ideas in the text which connect to my memory as a reader. Here I develop organizing ideas, which logically guide the construction of my personal response text. It is at this phase of my cognitive processing operation that I develop my sense of a rhetorical purpose in order to make meaning.